Amazing Brain and Body Breakthroughs

How to Enhance Your Memory, Avoid Alzheimer's and Improve Your Health and Thinking at Any Age

Publisher's Note

FC&A
103 Clover Green
Peachtree City, GA 30269

Produced by the staff of FC&A

First printing January 2001

ISBN 1-890957-47-X

Table of Contents

Introduction

In 1990, President George Bush and the United States Congress designated 1990-1999 the "Decade of the Brain." Few political declarations ever turned out to be so accurate. Scientists learned more about the brain in that decade than in all of human history.

Your brain only weighs about 3 pounds, but it's probably the most complex object on earth. It affects your every thought, movement, and emotion. Without it, you would simply not exist.

Yet, the importance of the brain has not always been recognized. About 2,500 years ago, the Greek physician Hippocrates, who is considered the father of modern medicine, was the first to theorize that the brain was the center of mental life. Greek philosopher and biologist Aristotle disagreed. He believed the heart was the source of human thought and emotion, and the brain was just an organ for cooling your blood. It took another 600 years for most scientists to decide that Hippocrates was correct.

Although it took hundreds of years for scientists to agree that mental abilities come from your brain, in less than 10 years, researchers uncovered an overwhelming amount of information about this small, wrinkled organ and how it works. Many of these discoveries will help doctors treat disorders of the mind. Others will help you keep your brain healthy and alert. Here are a few of the latest findings:

- With mental stimulation, your brain continues to grow new connections.

- Common anti-inflammatory drugs, like ibuprofen, may help prevent Alzheimer's.

- Exercise improves your mind, as well as your muscles.

- High blood pressure can cause your brain to shrink.

- Stress may interfere with the growth of new brain cells.

We have gathered the latest research to bring you new and exciting information about your brain — how it works, how to keep it healthy, and how to make the most of the brainpower God gave you.

Looking for ways to supercharge your memory? How about learning to sharpen your thinking, become more creative, or teach yourself some new mental tricks? You'll find it all in *Amazing Brain and Body Breakthroughs — How To Enhance Your Memory, Avoid Alzheimer's and Improve Your Health and Thinking at Any Age.*

Is someone you love suffering from Alzheimer's or depression? Find out how you can deal with these problems, or avoid getting them in the first place.

Don't forget to do the puzzles and quizzes included in each chapter. Experts say stretching your mental muscle with puzzles like these builds a sharper, healthier brain.

We hope you enjoy reading *Amazing Brain and Body Breakthroughs.* Use it to help you improve your most amazing organ — your brain.

Your amazing brain

Inside your brain

The nuts and bolts of your mind

Do you think computerized machines are smarter and more capable than you are? Think again. Your brain is more complex than the most sophisticated computer. That may be hard to believe when you know the incredible tasks that computers can perform, from calculating seemingly impossible math problems to guiding a spacecraft through space.

Computers do have some advantages over the human brain. Information rushes through computer circuits millions of times faster than it can travel through your body systems. However, most computers can only process information one step at a time, which is called serial processing. Your brain, on the other hand, constantly processes millions of pieces of unrelated information at the same time. Think of New York's Grand Central Station at rush hour, and you'll have a good idea of what your brain goes through every minute of the day. And much of it takes place without you even being aware of it.

For example, think about what goes on at the dinner table. Your brain may be figuring out how far you should reach to grasp a glass of iced tea, while at the same time recalling and fitting together words to form a conversation, *and* deciding whether the person you are talking to seems happy or sad. That's quite a lot to accomplish in a split-second!

And even in such simple tasks as distinguishing a word's meaning, the human mind dwarfs the most sophisticated computer. Only a person can tell if the word "spot" means a mark on your clothes, a place in line, or the ability to see someone in the distance. And if you've ever used the spellcheck feature on a computer, you know your brain is much better at deciding if another word for rabbit is "hare" or "hair."

Your brain vs. a computer

If you doubt that your brain could take on a computer, check out these two ads. You could tell the difference between them much more easily than the most advanced machine.

House for sale. 100-year-old beauty decorated with taste. Less clutter for owners to clean up. A great deal. Call today! Needs little work or maintenance money. Trapdoor drops into full basement from house. Roof skylights. Leakproof. Can be shown at any time. No house offers less problem. House can be viewed at your convenience.

House for sale. 100-year-old beauty decorated with tasteless clutter. For owners to clean up a great deal, call today! Needs little work or maintenance. Money trap. Door drops into full basement from house. Roof skylights leak. Proof can be shown at any time. No house offers less. Problem house can be viewed at your convenience.

Don't underestimate your brainpower

In the hustle and bustle of today's world, people have learned to count on the power of machines. You come home from a busy day, pop a dinner into the microwave, and settle in front of the television, remote control firmly in your grasp. The bell dings in the kitchen, indicating that your dinner is cooked; and you wish you had a robot maid, like Rosie from *The Jetsons*, to bring it to you. You think a robot would go along nicely with all the other modern gadgets and gizmos that make your life easier.

But so far, robots like Rosie haven't come along. Why not? Because, like the scarecrow from the *Wizard of Oz*, they don't have a brain. And no mere machine can come close to the power of the human brain for moving, talking, and making decisions. You, however, do have a brain, and learning to use it to its greatest advantage can make your life happier, healthier, and more fulfilling than a robot or any other machine ever could.

> *"If the human brain were so simple that we could understand it,*
> *we would be so simple that we couldn't."*
>
> — Emerson M. Pugh, quoted by George E. Pugh,
> *The Biological Origin of Human Values*

The mind/brain connection

"She has a mind of her own." That may seem like a silly phrase, because of course she has a mind of her own, everyone does. Nevertheless, many parents have spoken that phrase, partly with exasperation, partly with pride. The expression refers to someone who acts independently rather than blindly following everyone else. You should naturally be proud of having your own mind. Your mind is what sets you apart from everyone else — more than your age, color, religion, or outer appearance.

What's the connection between your mind and your brain? Your brain is a part of your body, but your mind is so much more than just another organ or limb. It is also much harder to define. In fact, if you look in the dictionary, you will find numerous definitions for the word "mind." Your mind includes your personality, your attitudes, opinions, and the way you think, feel, and perceive. Neuroscientists say your brain enables your mind; or your mind *is* what your brain *does*.

> *"When Nature her great masterpiece design'd,*
> *And fram'd her last, best work, the human mind..."*
>
> — Robert Burns

Take a peek at your brain

If you could peel back your skull and take a peek at your brain, you probably wouldn't be impressed. After all, it only weighs about 2-1/2 to 3 pounds, roughly the size of two large grapefruits. That's a pretty small percentage of your body, even though it uses about 20 percent of all the oxygen you inhale.

If you touched your brain, it would feel soft and spongy — sort of like a bowl of half-congealed gelatin. But it's not one solid lump of processing power. It has many different parts that work together to form one of the most powerful and mystifying objects in the world.

People have always been fascinated by the brain. In the early 1800s, a doctor named Franz Gall came up with a theory that different areas of the brain controlled different aspects of your mental abilities. He thought the parts of your brain that were more developed would appear as bumps on your skull.

He invented a practice he called phrenology, which involved "reading" the bumps on your skull in order to reveal your brain's abilities and your personality traits. Although Gall was wrong about the bumps, he was right in thinking that different parts of your brain are responsible for different functions.

Today, researchers are rapidly learning more about which areas of your brain control different abilities. This knowledge may someday help scientists learn how to control diseases that affect your brain, like Alzheimer's.

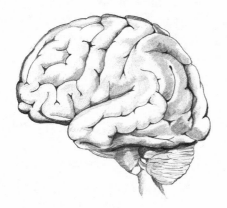

The human brain

The wrinkled gray surface of the brain may look like a mass of worms, but it is more complicated than the most advanced computer.

Your incredible cortex

You've probably heard the brain referred to as "gray matter." That's because the outer covering of your brain, the cortex, is grayish in color. The word cortex comes from the Latin word for "bark" because it resembles the bark of a tree. Only about one-third of it is visible; the rest lies within its wrinkled folds. If you could smooth out your cortex, it would cover an area about the size of a newspaper page or a pillowcase. Though your cortex is only about an eighth of an inch deep, it consists of around 30 billion nerve cells.

The cortex is only part of your brain, and it in turn is divided into sections, each responsible for different functions. Two narrow arch-shaped sections near the center of the cortex are called the sensory cortex and the motor cortex. When scientists probe these areas electrically, they can produce a response in another part of your body.

Motor cortex. The motor cortex controls muscle movement. This is the area from which your brain sends out messages to your body, telling it to move. By stimulating certain parts of the motor cortex with electricity, a scientist could make you smile, close your fist, or wiggle your toes, even against your will.

Sensory cortex. The sensory cortex is the area that receives information from your senses. When scientists stimulate different parts of this area of the brain, people report feelings of being touched in different parts of their bodies. They could feel a brush on the cheek or poke in the side even though the touches didn't actually occur.

Association areas. The sensory and motor portions account for only about 10 percent of your cortex. Sticking an electric probe into the rest of the cortex, called the association areas, doesn't produce any

Motor cortex   Sensory cortex

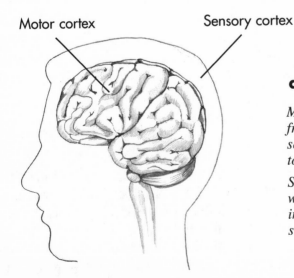

The motor cortex and sensory cortex

Motor cortex: the area from which your brain sends movement messages to your body.

Sensory cortex: the area in which your brain receives information from your senses.

reaction. This is probably the reason for one of the most popular misconceptions about your brain: that you only use about 10 percent of it. Scientists have long thought that if you could only tap into that unused 90 percent of your brain, you would become much smarter. However, they now know that area is already hard at work. It forms the workdesk area of your brain: organizing, interpreting, and making decisions based on information received from the sensory cortex.

Wrinkles you should welcome

Wrinkles around your eyes may indicate long hours spent squinting into the sun, or a lifetime of smiles; too much worrying may create wrinkles on your forehead. But what about the wrinkles in your brain?

One folksy explanation is that every time you learn something new, you create a new wrinkle. If that were true, however, some adventuresome people would have brains as wrinkled as slept-in clothes, while stuck-in-a-rut types would have brains as smooth as glass.

For the first six months in your mother's womb, your brain was indeed smooth. After that, it began to develop those interesting folds and wrinkles that make up the outside of the human brain. This wrinkling is the only way your body can fit the needed amount of brain matter into a space the size of your skull.

Scientists aren't sure how this happens. They think some brain cells may grow faster than others, or perhaps tension on parts of the cells distorts the cortex surface. However it happens, it's probably lucky for us that it does, because those folds contain lots of brain power.

You may not like wrinkles on your face, but wrinkles in your brain are a definite plus.

Get a feel for your emotional brain

Your brain is involved in much more than just thinking. It also plays a part in your emotions, motivations, and memories. A donut-shaped system inside your brain called the limbic system directs much of your emotional orchestra. Your limbic system consists of several structures that work together with hormones to influence your emotions.

Amygdala. You're alone on an unfamiliar street at night. You hear footsteps behind you. Does your heart start to race and your palms start to sweat? Do you quicken your step out of fear, or do you whirl around in anger, ready to confront your follower? Two little almond-shaped areas in your limbic system may affect your reaction.

Known as your amygdala, it influences aggression and fear. Experiments find that stimulating the amygdala can cause an animal to cower in fear or bristle with rage. The amygdala doesn't totally control these emotions, but it does play an important role, and understanding its function may someday help scientists understand how to control violent behavior.

Hypothalamus. It's a hot summer day, and you've been out working in your yard. You're feeling the heat, and visions of a tall, cool glass of lemonade are beginning to dance through your head. Another part of your limbic system may be responsible for that. Your hypothalamus regulates body temperature, hunger, and thirst. It also influences sexual behavior. Researchers find that certain areas of the hypothalamus are "pleasure centers" in animals as well as in humans. These centers are associated with the pleasures of eating, drinking, and sex.

Hippocampus. If you've ever watched a soap opera, you're probably familiar with amnesia. A character takes a sharp rap on the head and suddenly can't remember anything. Quite often another bump on the head or some emotionally upsetting event brings the character's memories flooding back.

Amnesia doesn't happen as often in real life as it does on soap operas. When it does, it usually involves damage to a part of your limbic system known as the hippocampus. This S-shaped structure plays a role in creating memories. An animal that has had its hippocampus removed cannot recall things learned in the preceding month or so but will retain older memories.

This implies that you don't store memories permanently in your hippocampus; it's more like a processing area where memories reside temporarily before being transferred to a permanent home elsewhere in your brain.

The limbic system: your 'emotional brain'

Hippocampus: involved in processing memories.

Amygdala: influences fear and aggression.

Hypothalamus: regulates hunger, thirst, body temperature, and sexual behavior.

Pituitary gland: part of the endocrine system rather than the brain, this master gland is influenced by the hypothalamus.

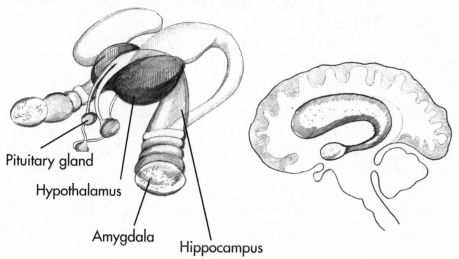

Pituitary gland

Hypothalamus

Amygdala   Hippocampus

Your master gland. At the base of your brain lies a pea-sized gland called the pituitary gland. Although it works closely with your brain, it is actually part of the endocrine system rather than your limbic system. Its close location makes communication with your brain easier and quicker.

Your hypothalamus sends signals to your pituitary gland, which in turn triggers other glands in your body to produce hormones. These hormones are chemicals that travel through your bloodstream and affect your mood and behavior. They also affect your brain, creating a circle of continuous communication between your brain and the rest of your body.

Lower brain keeps you going

Your "old brain." Your most basic functions of living, your breathing and your heartbeat, depend on the oldest area of your brain. Your brainstem begins where your spinal cord enters your skull and swells slightly, forming the medulla. All the nerves that run between the spinal cord and the brain pass through the medulla, and it is the "crossover" location for movement signals. The right side of your brain controls movement on the left side of your body, and the left side of your brain controls the right side of your body.

Your "little brain." If you can walk and chew gum at the same time, you have your cerebellum to thank. The name of this area at the base of your brain means "little brain." It looks like a smaller duplicate of the rest of your brain, wrinkled and divided in two halves. It plays a part in learning and memory, but its main function is to keep you moving along smoothly. If you injured your cerebellum, your movements would be jerky and awkward, and you would find it difficult to keep your balance.

When you are learning a new physical skill, skiing for instance, your cortex is in control. But once you learn that skill, your cerebellum takes over, and the movements become second nature. You no longer have to think "bend my knees, keep my back straight, look straight ahead," you just do it.

Your sensory switchboard. Whenever you touch, taste, hear, or smell something, that information passes through a brain region called the thalamus. This egg-shaped structure receives sensory input from nerve cells and directs it to various higher areas of your brain to be interpreted. It also receives some of the replies from those higher regions. Think of it as a type of neural train station where sensory input passes through en route to different destinations.

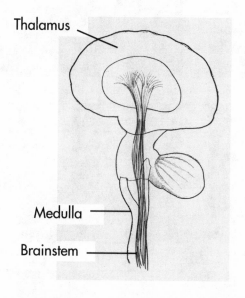

Thalamus

Medulla

Brainstem

The brainstem and thalamus

Brainstem: the oldest region of your brain.

Medulla: area of brainstem that controls breathing and heartbeat.

Thalamus: directs sensory information to other areas of the brain.

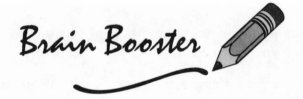

Cranial crossword

1	2	3		4		5					6	7	8		9	
10											11				12	
13			14								15					
		16			17							18	19	20	21
											22				
		23	24				25				26				
		27										28			
29	30												31		
32									33						
34			35		36						37		38		
39															
40															
41	42		43								44				
		45						46	47						
							48								
			49												
						50									

Across

1 _____ hath charms to soothe the savage breast.
5 Your amygdala plays a role in influencing feelings of fear and _____.
10 Intuition.
11 This kind of man didn't have a heart.
12 Not off.
13 Your brother's daughter.
15 Connecting word.
16 Not later
17 Touch someone, and the feeling is processed in their _____ cortex.
18 Brink.
22 Work for wages.
23 _____ disease occurs when you don't have enough of the neurotransmitter dopamine in your brain.
26 Word of frustration.
27 Not in.
28 The night before.
29 The wrinkled gray outer part of your brain.
31 Popular television show about doctors.
32 Facial blemish
34 Shakespearean king.
35 Where the "pleasure centers" of the brain are located.
39 Tom, Garfield, or Heathcliff
40 Suffix meaning "like."
41 _____ over; think about.
45 Your motor cortex controls _____ movement.
46 Desirable in your brain, but not on your face.
48 Male sheep.
49 Your brain is about the consistency of half-congealed _____.
50 Usually, a cat, dog, or bird.

Down

1 Your brain is the center of this type of activity.
2 "_____ it or lose it" applies to your brain as well as your muscles.
3 Twirl.
4 People who run the ship.
5 Damage to your hippocampus could result in _____.
6 Remain.
7 The wages of _____ are death.
8 A friend in need is a friend _____.
9 Not yes.
14 Your brain is more complex than the most sophisticated _____.
19 Challenge.
20 Serious.
21 Come in.
24 What you did with your supper.
25 Neurotransmitter targeted by many popular antidepressants.
27 Highly decorative.
29 Good for your bones.
30 Sea.
33 Your pituitary _____ works closely with your brain to help produce hormones.
35 Where your brain is.
36 Early "mind-reading" technique.
37 Your _____ is what your brain does.
38 Tiny gaps between brain cells.
42 The two halves of your brain are _____ by your corpus collosum.
43 System of brain structures that influences your emotions.
44 Speed _____.
46 Swaddle.
47 First-_____; top-notch.

Check your answers in the *Solutions to Brain boosters and teasers* section at the back of the book.

Chemicals spark communication

Your brain cells are nestled very close together, but there are tiny gaps between them called synapses. These cells must communicate across the synapses in order for you to move, think, or even breathe. This process is helped along by chemicals called neurotransmitters.

Researchers are finding that by helping your brain produce more or less of these important chemicals, you can battle brain disorders like depression, Alzheimer's, and Parkinson's.

Acetylcholine. One of the most important and abundant neurotransmitters is acetylcholine (ACh). It transmits messages between your brain and spinal cord and is involved in helping skeletal muscles move. Losing these nerve cells may be a factor in the development of Alzheimer's disease.

Serotonin. Not many prescription drugs have gotten as much publicity as the antidepressant Prozac. This drug works its wonders by making more serotonin available to your brain cells. The level of serotonin in your brain may affect your mood, your sleep habits, your sensitivity to pain, and your appetite.

Dopamine. This neurotransmitter plays a part in your muscle control and movement. Parkinson's disease, which results in tremors and loss of muscle control, may be caused by not enough dopamine in the brain. The main medicine used to treat Parkinson's, Levodopa, is meant to increase dopamine levels.

Norepinephrine. This chemical, like serotonin, may affect your mood and is the target of some types of antidepressants. It is also important in controlling your blood flow, heartbeat, and your response to stress.

Your divided brain

Two halves of a complex puzzle

It's the first day in a college classroom, and the professor is getting acquainted with his new students. He goes around the room one by one, asking students what their major is. "Accounting," answers one, and he makes a line on the left side of the blackboard. "Computer programming," answers another, and another mark goes on the left.

"Music," says someone, and a mark finally goes on the right side of the board. When everyone in the classroom has responded, the professor counts the marks on either side. There are four times as many marks on the left side as the right side.

"Do you know what this means?" the professor asks. "All these people ..." he circles the marks on the left side of the board, "are left-brained." He pauses and looks out at his classroom. "But this is a right-brained course, so most of you are going to need to pry open the right side of your brain and be more creative."

Left brain? Right brain? If you're like most people, you probably have no idea what the professor is talking about. Of course, when you have a tough time making a decision, you might feel as though you had two brains, each fighting for its own viewpoint. Well, you don't have two brains, but your brain is divided almost equally into two halves. These are called hemispheres and are connected by a wide band of nerve tissue known as the corpus collosum.

Researchers first became aware of the differences in these hemispheres through people who had brain injuries. They noticed that injuries to the left side of the brain resulted in different types of problems than injuries to the right side. Later they found that different areas of your brain actually perform different jobs.

For example, when a person speaks or does math problems, activity increases in the left side of his brain. That's why people who tend to be logical or analytical are known as "left-brained." When asked to solve a problem that involves perception, emotion, or creativity, activity increases in the right side of the brain. These types of people are called "right-brained."

So was the professor right? Can you classify people as right-brained or left-brained according to their interests? If you are a creative, emotional person, does that mean that only the right side of your brain is functioning? And if you are a logical, mathematically inclined person, does that mean you only use the left side of your brain?

Of course not. The two hemispheres of your brain work together, and your personality can't be explained that easily. But each side of your brain does control certain abilities, and researchers have pinpointed what these are.

"I am a brain Watson. The rest of me is a mere appendix."

— Sherlock Holmes in Sir Arthur Conan Doyle's
The Adventure of the Mazarin Stone

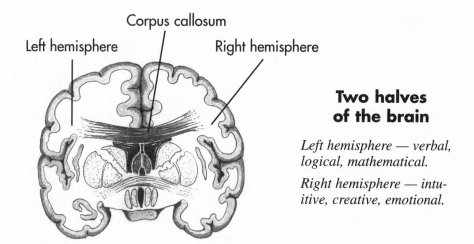

Corpus callosum

Left hemisphere

Right hemisphere

Two halves of the brain

Left hemisphere — verbal, logical, mathematical.

Right hemisphere — intuitive, creative, emotional.

Analyze problems with your logical 'left'

If you had a stroke that damaged the left side of your brain, you might end up with problems in reading, writing, and doing math. The stroke might also leave you paralyzed on the *right* side of your body. Damage to the right side of your brain would affect the left side of your body.

Because injuries to the left side of the brain resulted in such noticeable problems, doctors used to consider it your "dominant" hemisphere. Injuries to the right hemisphere weren't so obvious; but in recent years, doctors have discovered it is equally as important as the left. The left is dominant only in certain types of activities.

Logic. Whenever you look at a problem and analyze it methodically, your left hemisphere is probably hard at work. It is in charge of evaluating material in a logical manner.

Verbal ability. Your left hemisphere controls language skills. It affects your speech as well as your ability to read, write, and understand others.

Literal meanings. Your left hemisphere understands words, but only their most literal meanings. For example, suppose someone said to you, "I'd cut off my right arm for a piece of that cheesecake." Without your right hemisphere to interpret the exaggeration, your left brain would only understand the words themselves. It might actually believe your friend was willing to trade a vital limb for temporarily satisfying his sweet tooth.

Linear information. Organization rules in the left hemisphere. It processes information one step at a time, in sequence.

Mathematical ability. Like letters that make up words, the numbers and symbols that make up math problems are recognized by your left hemisphere. You also use the logical ability of your left brain to reason out and analyze math problems.

The 'right' way to worry

Some people worry about everything, while others seem to skip happily through life like Alfred E. Neumann (What? Me worry?). Whether you are an incurable "worry-wort" or just suffer occasional twinges of worry, a recent study finds it takes place in the right side of your brain.

Researchers asked volunteers to make tapes describing their worries. The volunteers were then asked to listen to the tapes. PET scans revealed more activity in the right frontal lobes when volunteers listened to their "worries" tapes than when they listened to neutral tapes.

This adds to evidence that the right side of the brain is more involved with emotions; worry occurs when the brain is unable to come up with a simple, logical solution to a problem, and emotion takes over.

Creativity — your right brain at work

If you injured the right side of your brain, you would probably be able to speak, but you might not understand what other people said to you. You might also have trouble finding your way around or fitting the pieces of a puzzle together.

Non-verbal understanding. The right side of your brain concentrates on images rather than words.

Spatial ability. Your right brain helps you figure out visual-spatial relationships. Whenever you're working a jigsaw puzzle, or figuring out which route to take on a trip, your right hemisphere is probably working hard.

Intuition. While the left side of your brain is concerned with logic and reality, your right brain commands your intuition and imagination. Your left brain might hear a noise downstairs at night, but it is your intuitive, imaginative right that tells you that noise may mean danger.

Figurative meanings. Your right brain interprets the meanings behind words. If a friend says to you, "He was pulling my leg," the right side of your brain helps you understand that means someone was teasing your friend, not actually pulling on her leg.

Overview information. While the left side of your brain processes information one piece at a time, your right brain views multiple pieces of information simultaneously, as a whole.

Emotions. Emotions actually come from the limbic system in your brain, but the right side of your brain is more in tune with your emotional state than your left side.

Is your cat a southpaw?

The most obvious evidence of your divided brain is your hand preference. Almost all people use one hand more than the other, with most people preferring their right hand.

This handedness isn't limited just to humans, however. Even animals use one paw more than the other. In studies, cats generally use just one paw when reaching for objects, and mice will reach for food with the same paw almost every time.

Hand preferences seem to be a natural occurrence, and you may not be that much different from Fido. However, animals have one big difference from humans in their paw preferences. About 50 percent of cats, monkeys, and mice favor their right limb over their left. About 90 percent of humans favor their right hand over their left.

Researchers tried breeding mice that shared the same paw preference for three generations, but they still came up with a 50/50 ratio of right-pawed and left-pawed mice.

Right-hand preference in humans may be related to the fact that language is controlled mostly by the left hemisphere, along with the right side of your body. Animals don't have language ability like people, so they may be less likely to favor the left side of their brain, and thus the right side of their body.

Good news for lefties

"If the right side of the brain controls the left side of the body, only left-handers are in their right mind."

This comment is emblazoned on tee shirts and bumper stickers, usually (if not always) displayed by left-handers tired of being put down for their difference. Left-handers have sometimes been considered strange; the word "sinister" comes from the Latin for "on the left."

Though far from being evil or sinister, the brains of left-handers do tend to be a little different than right-handers. Almost all right-handers process speech in the left hemisphere of their brains. More than half of left-handers also process speech in their left hemisphere, but some of them process it in the right hemisphere, and others use both hemispheres equally for speech. Since this probably requires better communication between the hemispheres, the corpus collosum, which connects the two hemispheres, is an average of 11 percent larger in left-handers.

About 10 percent of the population is left-handed. This preference for using one hand over the other begins before birth. Ultrasounds of fetuses in the womb reveal that more than 90 percent of them suck the right-hand thumb.

Several years ago, reports showed that left-handers lived an average of nine years less than right-handers. Luckily, new statistics find that isn't true. The statistics were skewed by parents who forced their naturally left-handed youngsters to become right-handed.

So if you are a left-hander, whether you're in your right mind or not, you can expect to live just as long as your right-handed neighbor.

Hidden clues to disease and illness

Any artist or craftsman will tell you the right tools make all the difference. It's difficult to carve a delicate trinket box with a chainsaw. Brain researchers would probably agree.

Early researchers could only examine the brains of dead people, or study people whose brains were damaged in some way. They had some idea of how the brain worked, but it was very general. Many of the modern breakthroughs in brain research involve high-tech ways to look inside the living brain for hidden clues to how it works.

Medical technology has come a long way since X-rays first allowed doctors to peer inside the human body without cutting it open. Although X-rays still have a place in diagnosing medical conditions like broken bones, other techniques provide doctors and scientists with more detailed images without the risks of radiation. Most of these techniques have long, tongue-twisting names, so they are usually referred to by initials.

CT (computerized tomography) scan — This method, developed in 1972 specifically to study the brain, combines X-rays with computer technology to produce more accurate images of your brain with less radiation. CT scans made the diagnosis and treatment of strokes, tumors, and brain injuries much easier. In 1982, this scanning method helped save the life of James Brady, President Reagan's press secretary, who had a bullet in his brain meant for the President. It is now used, not just for the brain, but for scanning other organs as well.

MRI (Magnetic resonance imaging) — In this method, powerful magnets provide images of your brain and other organs. An MRI can produce a detailed image that can reveal tumors or track blood flow. MRI works without radiation, which minimizes the danger of side effects. However, if you have a pacemaker, hearing aid, or other electrical device, the MRI could interfere with it.

EEG (Electroencephalogram) — Electrical impulses rush through your brain constantly. An EEG measures that electrical activity in your brain. It can show how much activity is going on, and by recording different patterns, help diagnose certain brain disorders, such as epilepsy.

PET (Positron emission tomography) scan — Your busy brain uses lots of fuel, mostly glucose. PET scans detect activity in different areas of your brain by measuring how much glucose is being consumed. This imaging method has been particularly helpful in pinpointing the areas your brain uses for different tasks.

These imaging techniques have provided scientists with wonderful tools to peer inside a living brain. They have helped them discover which parts of your brain control various activities, and have revealed hidden clues to disease and illness. One amazing discovery is that the brain is remarkably elastic, so much so that it can often reroute functions from damaged brain areas to healthy areas.

Thanks to these modern technological tools, we can now identify and treat diseases and illnesses much sooner than before. And that means a healthier future for all of us.

Brain Booster

Know your body

No bones about it, you should know as much as you can about your own body. See if you can answer these trivia questions about the human body.

1. What is by far your body's largest organ?
2. What organ contains the smallest bones?
3. What's the strongest muscle in your body?
4. Which of your senses becomes dulled when you eat too much?
5. If you've ever struck your funny bone, you know it doesn't make you laugh, so why is it called a funny bone?
6. Where's your coccyx?
7. Where on your body can you find 20 moons?
8. If you were struck by lightning, which of your senses would you be most likely to lose?
9. What do men have about 13,000 of?
10. Which of your five senses developed first?
11. What is the largest muscle in the human body?
12. What bodily function can occur at speeds of up to 200 miles per hour?
13. What are the four tastes?
14. What organ is affected by encephalitis?
15. Where in your body do you have lacrimal fluid?
16. What's the name of the punching-bag-type thing that dangles in the back of your mouth?
17. What bone is most often broken?
18. Which of your senses is most closely connected to your memory?
19. What is it impossible to keep open while sneezing?
20. How many bones are there in the human body?

Check your answers in the *Solutions to Brain boosters and teasers* section at the back of the book.

Male vs. female

Brain differences between the sexes

You wake up in the morning and hear birds warbling happily outside your window. Did you know that the birds you hear are almost all male? Male songbirds sing their happy tunes to attract females. And to perform these enticing concerts, they rely on their "music center," a portion of their brain that is about six times larger than in females. This difference in brain structure influences male and female songbirds to behave differently.

Most people agree that male and female humans also behave differently. Little boys generally prefer toy guns to Barbie dolls. Girls play dress-up and nurture their baby dolls. Many of these behavior differences may be accounted for by the way society, including parents, treats boys and girls differently.

Yet many mothers have discovered that they can refuse to buy their sons toy guns, giving them less violent toys instead, and they will still form them out of sticks, coathangers, or even their fingers. Surely, you think, as you watch a group of boys tousling on a playground while the girls play quietly with their dolls, their brains just work differently.

As it turns out, there are differences, although not nearly as obvious as in songbirds. If you could take a male and a female brain and put them side by side on a table, you probably couldn't tell which was which. However, internal differences do exist, and they may provide researchers with some pieces to the puzzle of why men and women behave differently.

Size — a difference you can ignore

Do you think bigger is always better? If most of the products in your pantry say giant-size, family-size, or huge economy-size, you probably do. If you're a scrupulous comparison shopper, however, you know that size can sometimes be deceiving.

Size accounts for one of the most controversial differences between the male and female brain. Male brains are an average of 10 to 15 percent larger than female brains. Some scientists argue that this shows men are more intelligent than women. Others disagree, arguing that males have bigger bodies, so the difference in brain size merely reflects the body size difference. Of course, the position that each scientist takes on this issue may be influenced by whether that scientist is male or female.

But for those men who think they're coming out on top in this debate, watch out. While male brains start out larger than women's, research has found they tend to lose brain tissue almost three times faster than women as they age, particularly in the regions relating to memory.

How can this shrinkage be prevented? C. Edward Coffey, of the Henry Ford Health System in Detroit, says one way is to limit alcohol intake, noting that too much alcohol makes the brain shrink faster. He also suggests watching your cardiovascular risk factors, particularly high blood pressure.

Dr. Ruben Gur believes the reason men's brains may shrink is because they overuse certain brain cells. In his study, PET scans monitored activity in people's brains while they performed a mental task. Then he asked the people to relax. When the women were asked to relax, PET scans revealed that they did turn their thoughts elsewhere.

However, when the men were asked to relax and think about something else, PET scans showed that the same brain cells remained at work, suggesting the men were still fixed on the task. This may result in overuse of brain cells, causing them to "burn out."

A good lesson to learn from Gur's research is to avoid stressing out over a particular problem. Force yourself to relax and turn your attention to something else. If you don't, you may just burn out the very cells you need to solve the problem. And shrink your brain in the process!

Survive your next road trip together

In a scene from the movie *Bridges of Madison County*, Meryl Streep tries to give Clint Eastwood directions to a bridge. After a few attempts to describe landmarks to him, she gives up and decides to just show him the way. This scene illustrates one of the brain differences between men and women — how they process certain information. It also shows how miscommunication often results from these differences.

Research finds that men and women learn certain tasks differently and excel at different types of tasks. And, just like Streep and Eastwood, one of the things they learn differently is how to find their way.

Unfortunately, if you're like most couples, these learning differences may have contributed to a major battle at some point in your travels together.

The problem is that men and women use different means to remember directions. Women tend to identify directions with landmarks. If you asked a woman for directions, she might tell you to turn left at the big oak tree, or right by the white house with green shutters.

Men seem to learn routes faster, but they can't recall landmarks as well as women. Instead, they rely on direction and distances. If you asked a man for directions, he might tell you to go about three miles east on Hwy. 134 and turn west on Ingles Road.

So if you try to give your husband directions in typical female fashion, he may have a difficult time following them.

Hormones apparently account for some of these differences. Studies find that female rats, like women, tend to learn maze routes by using landmarks such as pictures, while male rats rely on geometric cues like angles. If no landmarks are available, however, female rats will use geometric cues, but male rats still will not use landmarks.

However, if researchers adjust the levels of sex hormones like estrogen and testosterone during the rats' development, female rats behave like males and males behave like females.

So the next time your husband refuses to ask for directions or tries to find his way by "following his nose," try to be a bit more understanding. After all, he's just doing what his male brain tells him to.

"I'm not denyin' the women are foolish;
God Almighty made 'em to match the men."

— George Eliot

Follow the lead of London cabbies

Taxi drivers in big cities like London and New York are amazing. No matter how out-of-the-way your destination, they can take you straight to it. Do they have a map of the city etched on their brain?

Well, not exactly. But researchers in England have discovered something different in the brains of London cabbies. Their rear hippocampus — the zone associated with navigation and spatial memory — is much bigger than that of most people.

Could it be they were born that way and were hired as cab drivers because of their good sense of direction? No — the average taxi driver in London spends two years studying maps of the city before taking the test to get the required license.

And when researchers compared the brains of cabbies who started driving 40 years ago with those who started more recently, they found the rear hippocampus was much larger in the old-timers. The researchers think it was the years of driving the streets of London that caused the increase in size.

Practice, it seems, does make perfect. But if you are thinking about becoming a cab driver to improve your sense of direction, be aware you might have to give something up. The scientists learned that while the rear hippocampus of taxi drivers was larger, the front of the hippocampus was smaller than average. They aren't sure what that means because they don't know exactly what that part of the brain does.

Maximize your mental skills

How they learn directions (or whether they'll ask for directions) isn't the only difference in the way men and women learn tasks, or what kind of tasks they excel at. Men tend to be better at tasks that involve spatial relationships, mathematical reasoning, or hitting a target. This may be why men enjoy sports like basketball, baseball, or golf that require those types of abilities.

Women, on the other hand, tend to be better at tasks that involve verbal fluency, rapidly matching objects, mathematical calculations, or fine motor coordination.

If you want to keep your brain in top-notch shape and maximize its abilities, make sure you vary your mental workouts to include things you don't normally do. For example, if you enjoy word puzzles, like many women, try some math puzzles. Or maybe even challenge someone to a rousing game of darts to improve your targeting skills.

For men who love target games, why not relax and do a mind-bending crossword puzzle once in a while? Whether you're male or female, your brain will appreciate the extra challenges that come with learning something new and unfamiliar.

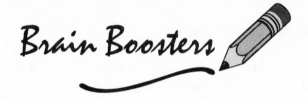

His and hers

Men and women excel at different types of problem solving, so here's a puzzle for each of you. Of course, you're welcome to try both for a little extra mental exercise!

Men can put their skills at solving spatial problems and understanding mathematical concepts to good use with the following two-part problem.

Question 1: Can you figure out how many running (linear, not square) yards of carpet you would need for this odd-shaped room? (See the following floor plan.)

Assume the carpet comes in widths of 12 feet. You'd like to lay it in one piece, without seams, even if you have to waste some carpet to do it.

Question 2: If the cost for the style you have selected is $20 a square yard, how much will you have to pay for your carpet?

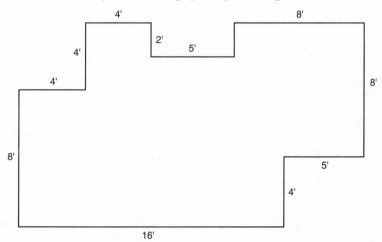

(If you are a male, you might want to have a female check your mathematical calculations before you head for the carpet store with your checkbook!)

Go to the *Solutions to Brain boosters and teasers* section at the back of the book to see if you've figured correctly.

Word maker

Women tend to do better at tasks that require verbal abilities. Look at this puzzle and try to make as many words of four letters or more as you can. In making each word, a letter must be used only once, unless it appears twice in the list. No plurals ending in "s"; no foreign words; no proper names. There is at least one nine-letter word contained in the list.

I   I   M

V   S   P

R   O   E

Compare your words to those in the *Solutions to Brain boosters and teasers* section at the back of the book.

Score:

20 words — good
30 words — very good
39 words — excellent

Intelligence

Maximize your mind's potential

Are you a "brain?" Brains and intelligence are sometimes thought of as practically the same thing. But let's face it, everyone has a brain. Everyone, however, is not considered intelligent or "brainy." What exactly is intelligence? What does it really have to do with your brain, and how much control, if any, do you have over it?

Defining intelligence is kind of like describing clouds. Everyone may agree on a partial description, such as white and fluffy, but some people see cotton balls where others see an alligator. Everyone also may agree on the basic concept of intelligence, but as far as what makes a person smart, forget it. There are as many opinions as there are people.

If you look in the dictionary, Webster's first definition of intelligence is "the ability to learn or understand from experience." According to this source, intelligence is the ability to learn, not how much you have learned.

Intelligence and knowledge may be related, but they are not the same thing. You don't necessarily have to be intelligent to acquire a lot of knowledge, although it certainly helps. The child who gets straight A's in school may be very intelligent or may just be persistent and hard-working. By the same token, some intelligent people may not have much knowledge, if they haven't had educational opportunities or if they have no ambition to learn.

The bottom line is, whether you are "brainy" or not, making the most of your intelligence can help you make the most of your life.

"Genius is 1 percent inspiration, 99 percent perspiration."

— Thomas Edison

How to be the smartest person in the world

If you read the Parade section of your Sunday newspaper, you may have seen a column written by "the smartest person in the world." Marilyn vos Savant holds this claim because she is listed in the *Guinness Book of World Records* as having the highest score ever on an intelligent quotient (IQ) test. But does that really make her the smartest person in the world?

Opinions differ on whether a test can accurately measure your intelligence. And no one can agree on exactly what intelligence is either, so a more appropriate title for Ms. Savant might be "the world's highest IQ score holder."

If IQ tests don't measure intelligence, well, what does? Perhaps an easier and better way to measure it is by life's successes, both personal and professional. In that case, who knows? Ms. Savant may indeed be the smartest person in the world. Or it could be your next-door neighbor. Or you.

IQ tests were invented to predict how students would perform in school so children with learning difficulties could be identified and receive extra help. Current intelligence tests compare your score to others your age, with a score of 100 being average. About 75 percent of the people score between 85 and 115.

Intelligence tests are generally good in predicting a person's range of ability, but a high score on an intelligence test doesn't mean you will breeze successfully through life. Also, if you took IQ tests on different days, your scores might vary by a few points for a number of reasons. You may or may not be good at taking tests. You may have had a headache when you took the test, or you may have been distracted by a personal problem.

A high score on an intelligence test is not a license to success and happiness. Many people with high IQ scores never achieve the level of success or happiness they would like. Many people with low IQ scores are highly successful and perfectly content. It's not how much intelligence you have, it's what you do with it that counts.

"Almost all the joyful things of life are outside the measure of IQ tests."
— Madeleine L'Engle, *A Circle of Quiet*, 1972

An easy way to beef up your brain

Do you owe your intelligence to your mother and father? Scientists not only disagree on the definition of intelligence, they disagree on where intelligence comes from. Is it determined by your genes or by your environment? This debate is often referred to as nature versus nurture.

Think about your brothers or sisters. Are you smarter than they are? You have the same parents, so you have many of the same genes.

Of course, unless you were adopted, you probably were also raised in the same environment.

So if you are smarter, is it because you got better genes from your parents or because they paid more attention to you as a child? Maybe it's just because your room was painted blue and your sister's was painted pink. You can see how confusing this issue can be.

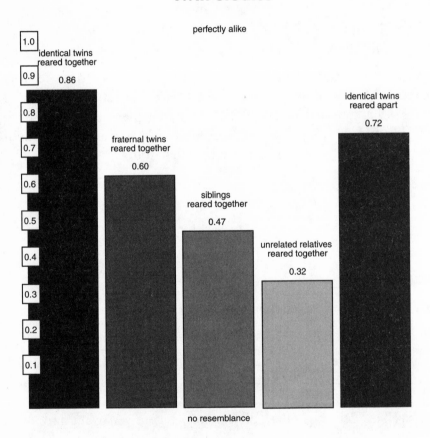

Twin studies

People who are the most genetically similar also have the most similar intelligence scores, although environment does play a role. (1.0 indicates a perfect correlation, while 0 indicates no correlation.)

Created by Thomas J. Bouchard, Jr., 1982

Identical twins who were separated at birth and adopted into different families shed some light on the dilemma of nature versus nurture. Although they have the same genes, they grew up in different environments, so researchers often study them for clues to intelligence and other traits.

According to studies, identical twins are more similar in intelligence than any other group. Even identical twins who were reared apart are much more similar than unrelated people who grew up together. This shows that heredity plays a greater role in determining intelligence than environment.

Does that mean your genes totally control intelligence, and there's nothing you can do to increase it? Not necessarily. Twins raised together are more similar in intelligence than twins reared apart, so environment must play some part. This would mean that you do have some control over your own intelligence. So give your brain lots to think about through a variety of rich cultural experiences, mental challenges, and interesting relationships. Go out and live an exciting life! By actively strengthening all areas of your mind, you'll be doing everything possible to enhance the intelligence you were born with.

Smarten up with mental workouts

In the cartoon *Pinky and the Brain*, the Brain is a mouse whose forehead bulges out noticeably. Obviously, his head can barely contain the large brain it must require to hold so much intelligence. Pinky's head, on the other hand, is rather small, appropriate for someone so dim-witted. Does bigger always mean better (even if you're not from Texas)? And does a bigger hat size indicate more intelligence?

Animals may provide a clue to this question. The brain of a whale is almost certainly bigger than the brain of a man, but in relation to its size, it is a mere pea-brain. A whale's brain only accounts for 1/10,000th of its weight, while the brain of a man accounts for 1/45th of his weight. Does this mean that the larger the brain in proportion to the body, the more intelligent the animal? Not always. The brain of a mouse is 1/40th of its body weight, but men are generally considered smarter than mice (even Mickey).

The answer seems to be that size does matter. However, what matters more is how much of the brain's size is devoted to association areas, where most of the "higher thinking" occurs. Animals usually have more of their cortex devoted to sensory areas, which is why they have such acute senses. We may not be able to smell something from a mile away like a coyote, or spot a tiny mouse from high up in the air like an eagle, but we can reason and think abstractly better than they can.

Brain size may also play a part in intelligence differences in people. Studies have found a slight correlation between brain size and intelligence in people. But what makes a brain larger? Is it simply heredity or can you increase the size of your brain, thereby raising your intelligence?

Animal studies find that rats who are raised in an enriched environment develop a thicker brain cortex. Like a body-builder who enlarges his muscles with exercise, perhaps you can enlarge your brain with mental work outs. Try reading, solving riddles, or learning a new skill. There are all kinds of ways to keep your mind in tip-top shape. Look for more suggestions in the chapter *Your aging brain*.

Revenge of the four-eyed nerd

Were you a bookworm who wore thick glasses in school? Were you ever called "four-eyes," or a "nerd" by the other kids? If so, take comfort in the fact that research shows that near-sighted people tend to be more intelligent.

One study found that not only did near-sighted students score higher on IQ tests, they also made generally better progress in school and had higher math grades than their eagle-eyed classmates.

7 ways to develop your own unique intelligence

You probably know someone who is "book smart" but has no common sense. You may also know people who are mechanically-inclined or brilliant musicians, but are not considered intelligent in the conventional sense.

If you browse bookstore shelves, you will quickly realize that the idea of other types of intelligence besides the kind measured by IQ tests is becoming more popular. In his book *Emotional Intelligence*, Daniel Goleman examines the fact that people with high IQ scores and perfect grades can still do very stupid things. He believes that emotional intelligence, which includes such qualities as self-awareness and control, persistence, motivation, empathy, and social skills, is much more important in dealing with life.

Other theories on multiple intelligences believe that everyone has their own type of intelligence, and if you know which type you possess, you can work to develop that area. You've heard of people who are "street smart." There are other kinds of "smarts" as well. Howard Gardner is credited with developing the first of this kind of theory. He has written several books on the subject, including *Frames of Mind: The Theory of Multiple Intelligences*, in which he describes seven types of intelligence. Decide which one (or ones) you are and then see what you can do to develop your own special intelligence.

Visual/Spatial Intelligence (Picture Smart) — Do you enjoy doing jigsaw or other visual puzzles? Do you like to draw or doodle? Can you see clear visual images when you close your eyes? Are you sensitive to color? If so, your area of intelligence may be visual-spatial. People in this category tend to become artists, architects, engineers, mechanics, and inventors. To make the most of your spatial intelligence: take classes in art or drafting, draw maps to familiar places, and improve your visual imagination by closing your eyes and picturing your favorite vacation spot, in as great detail as possible.

Musical Intelligence (Music Smart) — Can you tell if a musical note is off-key? Is listening to music an important part of your life? Do tunes often run through your head? You may have musical intelligence. Obviously, people with musical intelligence often become musicians — singing or playing an instrument. They might also become disc jockeys, composers, or choir directors. To use your musical intelligence to its fullest, fill your life with music. Listen to many different kinds of music to expand your mind. Experiment with different types of musical instruments.

Verbal Intelligence (Word Smart) — Do you enjoy word games like Scrabble? Are books very important to you? Were English, social studies, and history easier for you in school than math or science? If so, your area of intelligence may be verbal/linguistic. People in this category love words and tend to become writers, teachers, lawyers, and translators. To make the most of your verbal abilities, keep a daily journal, write a story, try to learn a new word every day and use it, and read as many different kinds of books as you can.

Logical/Mathematical Intelligence (Number Smart) — Can you easily solve math problems in your head? Do you look for patterns or logical sequences in things? Do you feel more comfortable when every-thing is measured, analyzed, or defined? You probably possess logi-cal/mathematical intelligence. People with this kind of intelligence usually become scientists, accountants, detectives, computer program-mers, and of course, mathematicians. Make the most of your intelligence by making up a logical explanation for something absurd or something you disagree with. Practice math skills by adding the price of items in the grocery store as you go along. Or set up "what if" experiments. For example, what if I use applesauce instead of butter in my muffin recipe?

Interpersonal Intelligence (People Smart) — Are you the kind of person others come to for advice? Do you enjoy teaching other peo-ple? Do you like to be involved in social activities through your church or community? Your strength may be interpersonal intelligence. People with this kind of intelligence are great communicators and tend to become counselors, political leaders, and teachers. To improve your interpersonal intelligence, volunteer in your community, practice focusing completely on what someone is saying, or try to guess what another person is thinking by their expressions and body language.

Intrapersonal Intelligence (Self-Smart) — Do you often spend time meditating or thinking deeply about your life decisions? Would you prefer an isolated weekend in a mountain cabin to a fancy party with lots of people? Do you keep a diary or journal? You may be particularly strong in intrapersonal intelligence. People with intrapersonal intelligence are very "in touch" with themselves and prefer to work alone. Therefore, many of them are self-employed. They also make good researchers. To make the most of your intrapersonal intelligence, practice yoga or meditation, and stop occasionally during the day to consider exactly what your inner feelings are at that moment.

Bodily/Kinesthetic (Body Smart) — Do you enjoy physical activity such as sports? Do you like working with your hands — making crafts or building things? Do you "talk with your hands," using gestures and hand movements to illustrate your point? Your intelligence may be in the bodily/kinesthetic area. These people tend to learn best by doing, and often become athletes, dancers, actors, and clowns. To use this type of intelligence to its fullest, play charades or other role-playing games; take up sports that use different types of skills, like golf and rowing; and practice being aware of how your body is moving as you do everyday chores like washing the dishes.

> *"We should take care not to make the intellect our god. It has,*
> *of course, powerful muscles, but no personality."*
>
> — Albert Einstein

Tips to turbo-charge your IQ

You may have your own type of intelligence, but you would still like to boost your overall IQ. A high score on an IQ test may not be a passport to success, but intelligence is a desirable quality, and you would like to improve that quality if you can.

One study on poor inner-city children showed that you can increase intelligence, at least at a young age. One group of children were provided with an enriched environment from the time they were infants. They were exposed to more learning opportunities, toys, playmates, and good nutrition. Another similar group of children were used as comparisons. When the children were 12 years old, researchers gave them IQ tests. The children who had grown up in the enriched environments scored significantly higher than the other children.

Whether adults can increase their intelligence that much is still a matter of debate, but research is discovering that some things may help you become smarter.

Music hath charms to raise your IQ. Music can be charming, soothing, or uplifting. It may also raise your IQ, but you have to listen to the right kind. One experiment had college students sit in silence or listen to Mozart or Muzak (elevator music) for 10 minutes before taking a standard IQ test. After the period of silence, the students scored an average of 110. After listening to Muzak, their average score was 111, not much of a difference. But after they listened to 10 minutes of a Mozart piano sonata, their average score jumped to 119.

Dr. Frances Rauscher, who performed the experiment, said that listening to complex kinds of music may stimulate neural pathways important in thinking. It may be kind of like warming up your car before you drive it. Simpler, more repetitive forms of music like Muzak may not provide the necessary level of stimulation.

The increase in intelligence may be temporary, but if you plan on taking a test or just need a little brain boost, put on some Bach or Mozart and get those brain cells fired up.

Bach for babies' brains

Zell Miller, former governor of Georgia, obviously cared about the education of children in his state. He was instrumental in starting the Hope Scholarship fund in Georgia, which has sent many students to college that may not otherwise have been able to go.

Because Gov. Miller cared about children's education, he also brought classical music to the babies of his state. Gov. Miller proposed that the state buy a cassette or CD of classical music to give to the parents of every baby born in Georgia. He cited the 'Mozart effect,' which showed that IQ scores increased after listening to classical music.

Whether or not you have a baby in your household, playing classical music may be an easy and pleasant way to increase your brainpower. If a state governor believes it, why shouldn't you?

The benefits of teaching. Have you ever thought you knew how to do something until you were asked to explain it to someone else? In the process of explaining it, you were forced to think more deeply about the subject and gained a better understanding of it yourself.

Research finds that birth order may affect intelligence levels, with the firstborn often scoring higher on tests than the following children. The lower on the birth-order ladder you are, the lower you are likely to score on IQ tests. You have no control over when your parents chose to have you, or how many siblings they chose to bless you with. But experts say that the reason the firstborn seems to be smartest is partly because he has the opportunity to "teach" his younger siblings. If you are an only child, you are always "last-born" because you were never given the opportunity to teach a younger sibling.

You don't have to be a professional teacher, or even a first-born child, to benefit from the experience of teaching. Teaching opportunities are all around you. Volunteer to teach reading to illiterate adults, or help out at your neighborhood school. Do you have a hobby — quilting, model-building, or rebuilding old motors? Take the time to explain your hobby to anyone who seems interested. You might just learn something yourself.

"I think, therefore I am."

— Descartes

'Smart drugs' may not be a smart move

You've probably seen the commercial. A man holds an egg and says, "This is your brain." Then he cracks the egg into a frying pan and says, "This is your brain on drugs." The sizzling egg paints a pretty scary image of frying your brain cells with drugs. It's almost enough to make you think twice before taking an aspirin.

On the other hand, the search for a drug that can make you effortlessly more intelligent is almost as pressing as the search for a drug that can make you effortlessly thin. "Smart drugs" are popping up everywhere. You can even buy "smart drinks," concoctions that are supposed to give your brain a boost. Smart drugs are particularly popular with many students, who take them before tests.

Smart drugs are also called nootropics, from the Greek for "acting on the mind." Some nootropics aren't drugs at all; some are herbs or nutritional supplements. Many are used to treat people with mental problems or diseases, but that doesn't necessarily mean they will help a normal, healthy person become smarter.

Before you pop a pill to improve your mind, check out some of the most popular ingredients in "smart drugs."

Hormones. Hormones may help make you smarter. Recent studies find that estrogen replacement therapy can help improve memory and maybe even help prevent Alzheimer's. Testosterone, that manly hormone, may also play a role in brain function. These hormones are available only by prescription.

DHEA, which may be converted into other hormones in your body, may also help you think faster. Your brain contains more DHEA than any other part of your body. Studies find that people with Alzheimer's have almost 50 percent less DHEA than people who don't have this disease. DHEA is available without a prescription, but some people experience side effects, which include excess hair growth in women, acne, mood swings, and fatigue. In addition, some doctors are concerned that it may also damage the liver, ovaries, prostate, or uterus.

The most effective hormone for your brain, however, may be something called pregnenolone sulfate. Pregnenolone helps your brain cells communicate. Studies find that this can significantly improve your ability to learn.

If you don't want to take prescription hormones, and you're uneasy about the side effects of over-the-counter hormones, you have another choice. Sleep on it. Taking a nap helps you boost those mind-improving hormones naturally; and it's cheap, easy, and safe. Not getting enough sleep can affect your levels of important hormones and neurohormones like pregnenolone. This may harm your ability to store information in your long-term memory.

Stimulants. Do you talk faster when you've had some caffeine? You may think faster, too. Studies find that stimulants like caffeine may increase your concentration and speed up your thought processes. Ritalin, a drug often used to help children concentrate in school, works this way.

Surprisingly, recent studies find that nicotine may have a positive side effect. Although it's long been considered an addictive, toxic substance, it also seems to enhance mental performance. Don't rush out to buy cigarettes in hopes of becoming the next Einstein, though. Stimulants only affect your short-term memory; they don't improve long-term recall. And the health risks of cigarettes definitely outweigh the temporary mental benefits.

But who knows? Someday, after more research has been done, nicotine just may be among the stimulants used to treat mental disorders or protect against memory loss.

Antidepressants. The connection between mood and mind is a close one. Studies find that people are better able to remember material when they are in a good mood. Antidepressants might help your mind by improving your mood.

In addition, animal studies are finding that antidepressants improve memory and learning skills. In one study, mice that had an antidepressant in their drinking water took much longer to show signs of age-related memory loss. The mice gained an equivalent of five to 10 human years of good memory. Human studies need to be done to confirm these findings, but improved learning may be an added benefit to antidepressant therapy.

Fatty acids. You've probably heard that fish is brain food. That's probably because it contains Omega-3 fatty acids, which help promote blood flow to the brain. Research has recently discovered that another fatty acid, phosphatidylserine, may also aid your brain.

Phosphatidylserine is a phospholipid, a fatty acid that is involved in communication between cells. Several studies have found that phosphatidylserine improves cognitive processes, especially in people who are significantly memory-impaired. One small study on depressed elderly women found that phosphatidylserine improved their mood, memory, and behavior.

Herbs. The grand-daddy of smart drugs isn't a drug at all, but rather an ancient herb. Ginkgo has been used for centuries to help brains function better. This herb improves blood circulation to your brain and is included in many nootropic formulas at your health food store. See the *Memory* chapter for information on this helpful herb.

Amino acids. Bodybuilders have long taken amino acid supplements to help build muscles. Today, many smart drug formulas you see in health food stores use amino acids as a base. Your body needs amino acids to build neurotransmitters, which carry messages between nerve cells in your brain. See the *Nutrition* chapter for details.

Vitamins. A deficiency of certain vitamins can cause mental problems, so will taking extra vitamins make you smarter? Probably not, but many smart drug formulas contain vitamins, especially B vitamins. However, if you aren't getting enough of these vitamins in your diet, you may indeed increase your brain power. The *Nutrition* chapter can tell you more about the importance of vitamins to your brain.

Choline. This is another popular ingredient in nootropics sold in health food stores. Your body needs choline to manufacture acetylcholine, a neurotransmitter important to learning and memory.

Some nootropics aren't available in the United States because they don't meet FDA approval. While you may be able to buy these through the mail, the FDA warns that drugs imported into the U.S. often do not meet the quality control standards of this country.

Will taking a smart drug turn a dull dud into a brilliant success? Don't count on it, but researchers continue the quest for safe and effective nootropics. In the meantime, if you choose to try smart drugs, be smart about buying them. Consult your doctor, read labels carefully, and buy from reputable companies.

The pH of IQ

When you were in school, your science teacher probably had you dip litmus paper into different solutions to see if it would turn red or blue. The color of the paper told you about the pH of the solution — whether it was more acid or alkaline.

Scientists in England have discovered that the pH of your brain may indicate how intelligent you are. Since you can't dip litmus paper into your brain, they used MRS (magnetic resonance spectroscopy) to study the brains of British schoolboys. They discovered that the more intelligent lads had brains that were more alkaline. Researchers speculate that alkaline brains allow nerve impulses to move faster.

Shampoos and skin creams may be able to balance the pH of your skin and hair, but you have no control over the pH of your brain. However, this research presents the fascinating future possibility of being able to raise your IQ by altering the pH of your brain.

Someday you may be able to turn your intelligence litmus paper from dumbbell red to genius blue.

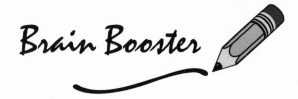

Brain Booster

'A' is for alphabet

Examine the following lines and identify what each letter stands for.

Example: 26 L of the A = 26 Letters of the Alphabet

1. 7 W of the A W
2. 1,001 A N
3. 12 S of the Z
4. 54 C in a D (with the Js)
5. 9 P in the S S
6. 88 P K
7. 13 S on the A F
8. 32 D F at which W F
9. 18 H on a G C
10. 90 D in a R A
11. 200 D for P G in M
12. 8 S on a S S

13. 3 B M (S H T R)
14. 4 Q in a G
15. 24 H in a D
16. 1 W on a U
17. 5 D in a Z C
18. 57 H V
19. 11 P on a F T
20. 1,000 W that a P is W
21. 29 D in F in a L Y
22. 64 S on a C
23. 40 D and N of the G F

Visit the *Puzzle Depot* Web site at <www.puzzledepot.com> for more trivia and puzzles.

Check your answers in the *Solutions to Brain boosters and teasers* section at the back of the book.

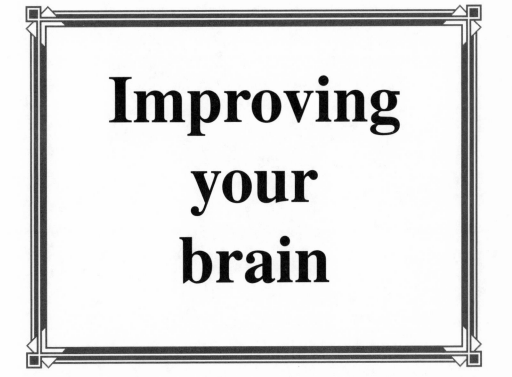

Improving your brain

Memory

Keys to recalling it all

Larry Benson cooked at a busy restaurant. All day long the waitresses would call orders in over a microphone, and then hang the tickets on a wheel for Larry to read. Larry rarely made mistakes on orders; until one day, the microphone broke. The waitresses couldn't call their orders in, so they just hung the tickets for Larry to look at.

The problem was, Larry had never learned to read. He was embarrassed to admit this to his employers, so he had depended on his memory to help him keep his job, remembering the details of dozens of orders at once.

This may seem a pretty amazing feat to someone who can't remember to fill their gas tank or turn the iron off. Larry became a memory whiz out of necessity, which proves what your brain can do when it has to. You may never need to have a memory like Larry, but almost everyone would like to improve their memory skills. Knowing how this complicated process works may help.

Your brain's personal photo album

Your brain contains so many memories, you could never count them all. Some memories are formed without any real effort on your part. You might remember a wreck you saw on your way home without even trying (or even while trying not to).

Other memories require a little more work. Remembering information for a test or a grocery list may require rehearsal. Almost everyone has walked to the store muttering something like "Bread, milk, butter, eggs, bread, milk, eggs, butter, bread..." Then a squirrel runs across your path, distracting you. You watch it for a moment, then resume chanting. "Bread, milk, butter ... What was that other thing?" Distractions can prevent you from forming a memory, which is why students should find a quiet study room.

Flashbulb memories. What were you doing when you heard the news of JFK's assassination or the Challenger explosion? Moments of strong emotion can cause memories to stamp themselves vividly into your brain. These are called flashbulb memories, because they occur as if your brain said, "This is important. Take a picture of it and save it." The reason your brain remembers these events so well is partly because of chemicals that flood the brain when your emotions are high.

The art of forgetting. As much as your brain is capable of remembering, it forgets much more. Every day you are bombarded with potential memories. People who have incredibly detailed and accurate memories may have more difficulty dealing with everyday problems, because they are constantly distracted by their many memories. Sometimes the ability to forget is as helpful as the ability to remember. Forgetting may come in handy, particularly when no one in the house wants to admit eating the last cookie.

Remembering the most important things may be the key to an ideal memory. For example, you can recognize a penny, but can you remember if Lincoln is facing right or left? It doesn't really matter as long as you know it's a penny. Your brain automatically sifts through the trivial to remember the important.

From short-term to long-term. Your brain handles two types of memory — short-term, or working memory, and long-term memory. Your short-term memory has a limited storage capacity. It can hold seven pieces of information, give or take two. The length of time you can hold information in your short-term memory varies from person to person. Do you look at a phone number in a phone book, and forget it before you finish dialing and have to look again, or can you look at a number in a phone book, walk down a hall, and dial it with confidence?

Regardless of how long your short-term memory is, your brain transfers some of that information into long-term memory. Unlike short-term memory, the amount of information you can store in long-term memory is virtually limitless.

Probing for memories. Once a memory has been transferred from short-term to long-term memory, you must be able to pull it out when you need it. Memories are stored in your brain like coat hangers in a closet, with some memories attached to others. Sometimes you have to pull out several "coat hangers" before you reach the one you want.

For example, you can't remember where you left your keys, so you retrace your steps. You walked in the front door, then you went into the kitchen, opened the refrigerator door ... Aha! You left them on the counter beside the refrigerator.

Sometimes the coathangers come flying out of the closet with no effort. You're standing in the grocery store, and an elderly woman walks by who wears the same perfume your great-grandmother wore. The smell instantly triggers a series of memories from family dinners to dominoes in the parlor.

Unfortunately, your coathangers sometimes get all tangled up on the floor of the closet, and you just can't find the one you want. Then, a memory is lost forever.

> *"No memory is ever alone; it's at the end of a trail of memories,*
> *a dozen trails that each have their own associations."*
>
> — Louis L'Amour

Tricks for a masterful memory

You could have sworn you put the title to your car in your safety deposit box, but it's not there. You witness a purse-snatching, and you are certain the criminal had shocking-blond hair, but another witness is equally certain he was brunette.

Sometimes you think your memory plays tricks on you. It happens to everyone, and it's OK, because you can also play tricks on your memory to get the most efficient and reliable use out of it.

People have been using memory tricks, called mnemonics for centuries. Ancient Greek and Roman orators remembered speeches by using a trick called the method of loci (location). They would associate each part of the speech with a part of their homes. For example, to recall the introduction to their speech, they would picture the entrance to their house.

Ancient Greeks aren't the only ones to boost their memories with mnemonics. If you learned "thirty days hath September" to remember how many days are in a month, or "every good boy does fine" for a piano scale, you've used mnemonics. Learning more about mnemonics can help you remember almost anything.

A few techniques apply to almost all methods of mnemonics:

Use all your senses. If you really want to remember something, make use of all your senses. Your brain has different types of memories, like visual memory and auditory memory. One of the most effective types of memory is olfactory memory, which involves your sense of smell. If you want to remember a moment, think about how the room looked, the sounds you heard, and what you may have smelled or touched. Remembering how something looked or smelled may trigger another memory, helping you get to the information you were looking for.

Make it vivid. Many methods of mnemonics involve visualizing something. You will remember it better if the memory is vivid, with bright colors and strong smells.

Make it funny. Everyone likes to laugh. When practicing your visualization, use humor. You will remember a funny image much better than a boring, everyday image.

Make it meaningful to you. When using association to remember something, try to relate it to your own life. For example, notice that someone has the same name as a relative of yours, or that a telephone number begins with the numbers of your birthdate.

Memory experts use mnemonic methods for remembering the most common things people forget. Ordinary people often use mnemonics too, usually without even knowing it. See if you have ever used any of the following memory techniques.

6 steps to perfect name recall

You hear your name called from behind you, and turn around to a familiar face. However, you can't remember the person's name. To most people, this is one of the most embarrassing memory lapses. Experienced salesmen know that people like it when you recall their names, so they have tricks for remembering.

Pay attention. The first rule is to focus on what it is you want to remember later. You already know it makes people feel special when you remember their names, so listen closely when someone introduces himself. Also, look directly at the person so you don't have any visual distractions.

Repeat it. After someone tells you his name, repeat it. "Nice to meet you, Steven." Saying the name impresses it into your memory better than just hearing it.

Spell it. If you think you need more reinforcement, ask him about the correct spelling of his name. For example: "Is that S-t-e-v-e-n or S-t-e-p-h-e-n?"

Comment on it. "Lilah, what a lovely name. My favorite aunt was named Lilah."

Associate it. Some names can be associated with something about the person. For example, you may think Lilah smells like lilacs, or Julie is wearing an interesting jewel on a necklace.

Use it. Once you know someone's name, use it often in your conversation to keep it fixed in your mind.

Remember, even with memory, practice makes perfect. The more you use these tips, the easier it will become. Go to a social gathering and practice your memory skills on the new people you meet. You'll not only make new friends, you'll make them feel special by remembering all their names.

Focus on faces

Some people pride themselves on never forgetting a face. Now, researchers have discovered that the brain has a special system for remembering faces. And it is separate from the one that helps you remember objects like trees and signposts.

Researchers recently studied a man who had suffered brain damage from a head injury. This man had difficulty recognizing ordinary objects like forks and chairs. But he could recognize faces even when researchers disguised them with wigs, glasses, or mustaches. He also could pick out caricatures of famous people, cartoon characters, and even faces made out of food.

Researchers believe this unique brain system works together with the one that recognizes objects to give you a complete picture of the world.

Lists — a powerful memory aid

You're standing at the grocery store with an empty cart. You've made a detailed list of everything you need, but as you fish through your pockets, you realize you forgot to bring it with you. Can you remember what was on that list?

The ability to remember lists is an important skill. One of the first things you learned in school was your alphabet, which is the foundation for reading. But at the time it was just a list of letters. You've learned other lists throughout your life — days of the week, months of the year, states, and capitols. Memory experts have several methods for remembering lists.

Take a journey. The journey method comes from the ancient Greek method of loci. Use a path you take daily, through familiar surroundings, like the path from your front door to your bedroom.

For example, if you need to remember a list of bread, milk, butter, and eggs, start by picturing your front door as a giant slice of bread with a knocker on it. Then move in your mind into the hallway and picture yourself wading through milk up to your ankles. Wade through the milk into your living room, and picture all the furniture smeared with butter, so that you would slide off if you tried to sit down. Next move into your bedroom, and picture a giant, egg-shaped bed. Now go to the grocery store, and to recall your list, just take a walk through your house.

Memory experts say that the more ridiculous you make your images, the more likely you are to remember them. Do you really think you could forget an image of yourself sliding off your butter-covered furniture?

Tell a story. The link method connects the items in your list together, usually by telling a story. Say you want to remember the names of the Great Lakes. Make up a story using the names of the lakes, or words that remind you of the names. Again, the more ridiculous the images in your story, the more likely you are to remember them. For example: SUPERman (Superior) was flying over the state of

MICHIGAN. A HERON (Huron) was standing near a lake below, his legs stuck ON a TAR-paved (Ontario) road. Superman swooped down and saved the heron, giving him an EeRIE (Erie) feeling.

Use some rhythm. One of the first lists you learned was your ABCs. And you were probably helped by the little song you learned along with it. Give your list a sing-songy rhythm, and it will be easier to remember.

Number chunking — Easy as 1, 2, 3

Your life is filled with numbers — phone numbers, social security numbers, credit card numbers, and driver's license numbers. Yet most memory experts agree that remembering numbers is their most difficult task. It's tough to assign meaning to a number, or use visualization.

When you have to remember long numbers like a phone number, you probably use chunking. Your short-term memory can hold only about seven items (like a telephone number), but by chunking numbers together, you can turn those seven items into two or three. For example, instead of trying to remember the number 1-4-3-1-9-8-5, think of it as one-forty-three; nineteen-eighty-five. Suddenly seven items are reduced to two easily remembered ones.

How to beat the 'lost again' blues

In a famous nursery rhyme, Little Bo Peep lost her sheep. Are you like this legendary lass, losing something every time you turn around? Luckily for her, the sheep showed up on their own. Your glasses, keys, and other lost items probably won't do that, so here are some tips to help you find them.

Put it in its place. If you have a problem remembering where you put things — your keys, for example — try to put them in the same place every time. If you make a habit of hanging your keys on a hook beside your front door, you won't spend frustrating mornings searching for them and ending up late for work. What else do you misplace on a regular basis? Your glasses? Your pen? Find a place for these items, and tell yourself, "Every time I put this down, I'm going to put it right here."

Retrace your steps. Occasionally, you'll slip up and forget to put an item in its place. Then it helps to retrace your steps. Try to remember the last time you used the item, and search from that point. For example, you know you used your keys to drive home, so start from your car and work your way into your house until you find them.

Visualize it. You can retrace your steps in your mind, or physically walk back over your path. Sometimes the sight of one item will trigger a memory about another item. Close your eyes and picture the item and where you were the last time you used it.

Remembering the 'write' stuff

No matter how hard you work on your memory, everyone forgets sometimes. The most helpful solution of all may be to write it down.

Keep a calendar by your phone so you can write down appointments as soon as you make them, and don't be embarrassed to use sticky notes around the house. A note saying "Take out the garbage" on your front door might draw snickers from your family, but it's worth it if it keeps the garbage from piling up.

Written reminders can come in handy, and sometimes just the act of writing something down will reinforce it in your mind. Then you won't even have to look at your "cheat sheet."

Rx for an ailing memory

Do you ever walk into a room and forget why you're there? Has anyone ever asked for your telephone number, and you just couldn't remember it?

Everyone has trouble remembering now and then. It doesn't necessarily mean anything is wrong with you. However, it can be annoying and sometimes embarrassing. You can use memory tricks to remember specific information, but you can also improve your overall memory with little effort. Research has discovered natural ways to help you do this.

A daily dose of help. If trying to remember your grocery list gives you a headache, you might reach for some aspirin. If you took the aspirin daily, however, you might remember that list more easily. Research finds that a daily dose of aspirin or other non-steroidal anti-inflammatory drug (NSAID) like ibuprofen can help you keep your mind sharp. It may even help you sidestep Alzheimer's disease.

A sweet memory jogger. A spoonful of sugar helps the medicine go down, according to Mary Poppins. According to research, a spoonful of sugar may help you remember to take your medicine. One study had people fast overnight, then gave them lemonade that had been sweetened either with sugar or a sugar substitute. Those who got the lemonade with sugar performed much better at a memory test than those who got the fake sugar, even the following day.

Does this mean you should fill your cabinets with candy bars and cakes to help you remember where you left your keys? Probably not; in this case, more isn't necessarily better. Although a lack of sugar may make you forgetful, too much is bad for your teeth and your waistline. Keeping your sugar level in balance may be what you need to be smart *and* healthy.

A colorful solution. Keeping your memories may be as simple as crunching some carrots. A recent study found that beta carotene, a substance found in carrots and other brightly colored fruits and vegetables, may help protect you from memory loss and other forms of mental impairment.

Researchers studied more than 5,000 people ages 55 to 95. They found that those people whose diets included the most beta carotene were the least likely to have problems with memory, attention span, and other mental abilities.

But if you despise carrots, don't despair. You can also get beta carotene in dark green vegetables like spinach and broccoli; and in yellow or orange fruits and vegetables like apricots and sweet potatoes.

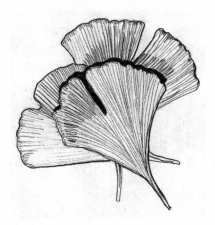

Ginkgo leaves

The fan-shaped leaves of the ancient ginkgo tree may help preserve your memories.

Miracle herb keeps memories alive

You may be able to leave your memory problems behind with the help of an ancient tree. The ginkgo tree, also known as the maidenhair tree, is the oldest living species of tree. The ginkgo was considered sacred in China, where monks helped keep this plant flourishing for centuries. Doctors in Europe write millions of prescriptions for ginkgo every year.

Ginkgo may help your memory by speeding up the blood flow to your brain. Your brain needs lots of oxygen to work properly, and your blood carries that oxygen.

Research finds that ginkgo widens your blood vessels so more blood can get through. It also helps make your blood less sticky, so it flows smoothly along. All this adds up to more blood flow and better short-term memory.

One study on men with age-related memory loss found that ginkgo supplements increased the speed at which their brains processed information taken in by their eyes. Other studies have shown that ginkgo improves the symptoms of cerebral insufficiency, such as lack of concentration and energy, confusion, absent-mindedness, anxiety, dizziness, and headache.

If you want to try ginkgo, it is available at health food stores as well as many grocery and drug stores. Most memory studies used a dose of 40 mg three times a day. Look for the words "50:1 concentrate" and "tannin-free" on the label. The 50:1 means that 50 pounds of leaves were used to make one pound of extract, which is the most effective ratio. Tannins are potentially toxic substances that are also found in ginkgo leaves, and should be removed during processing.

According to one source, the ginkgo tree was the only living thing to survive the bomb at Hiroshima. How appropriate that a plant so hardy may help you keep your memories alive a little longer.

Hormones help fight off forgetfulness

"Raging hormones" sometimes get a bad reputation for causing poor behavior in both men and women, but new studies find some hormones may improve your memory.

Estrogen replacement therapy (ERT) has long been recommended for women to ease symptoms of menopause. Then researchers discovered that ERT also seemed to protect women against heart disease. Now research has found yet another benefit to this hormone. Estrogen improves memory and may even protect against Alzheimer's.

One study found that women who were taking an estrogen-suppressing drug for fibroid tumors experienced a drop in their verbal memory scores. Scores improved in women who then received ERT to replenish their estrogen levels, but not in the women who didn't get ERT. Another study found that women who took ERT were one-third less likely to develop Alzheimer's than women who did not.

Women aren't the only ones to benefit from a memory-improving hormone. A recent study found that older men who were given testosterone supplements improved their working memories as well.

Hidden cause of memory loss

Have you always been known for your great memory that now suddenly seems to be slipping? Are you worried that it's the beginning of Alzheimer's? Before you panic, check your medicine cabinet. The answers to your memory questions may be in there.

Some medications can cause memory loss. Check your labels to see if you're taking any of the following medicines. If so, talk to your doctor about your memory loss, and ask if you can try another medication.

Don't discontinue taking prescription medicine without asking your doctor. Many of the drugs listed are for serious conditions, and a little memory loss may be a small price to pay to control that condition.

- High blood pressure — methyldopa, metoprolol, nifedipine, and propranolol.

- Cold and allergy — containing: brompheniramine, cephalexin, ciprofloxacin, diphenhydramine, metronidazole, ofloxacin, pseudoephedrine.

- Anti-depressants, anti-anxiety and insomnia — phenobarbital, alprazolam, amitriptyline, butabarbital, desipramine, diazepam, imipramine, lorazepam, nortriptyline.

- Heart disease — digoxin, disopyramide, quinidine, tocainide.

- Ulcer — cimetidine, ranitidine, famotidine.

- Arthritis — hydrocortisone, prednisone, cyclosporine, baclofen, cyclobenzaprine, indomethacin, methocarbimol.

- Pain and nausea — hydrocodone, meperidine, metoclopramide, oxycodone, prochlorperazine, promethazine.

- Parkinson's — levodopa, bromocryptine, pergolide.

4 can't-miss memory boosters

Move it or lose it. If you lose your glasses four or five times a day, perhaps you shouldn't move them around so much. Or perhaps you should move yourself around more.

Research finds that exercise can give your brainpower a boost. Exercise increases the blood flow to your brain, feeding it with oxygen and nutrients. Exercise also increases brain chemicals that help the growth of new brain nerve cells. Another brain benefit of exercise is that it helps control high blood pressure, which may actually cause your brain to shrink. If you exercise regularly, you can have it all — brains and brawn.

Break the stress cycle. Cutting stress from your life completely may be an impossible task, but if you value your memories, you should at least try to control your stress level.

Research finds that extreme stress causes your hippocampus to shrink. This is the part of your brain most closely involved with memory. A study of Vietnam vets with post-traumatic stress syndrome found that those who spent more time in combat had significantly smaller hippocampuses.

This is probably because hormones like adrenaline and cortisol are released during times of great stress. Those hormones help engrave "flashbulb memories" into your brain, but too much of them over time can cause damage.

You may not have the stress level of a soldier in combat, but controlling your stress may help you hold onto your pleasant memories a little longer.

Don't let your memories go up in smoke. Can't remember where you left your cigarettes? That's one thing you probably should forget. Experts have long believed that smoking contributes to diminished brain function by decreasing oxygen to your brain.

A recent study of 3,000 elderly men adds evidence to this belief. Men who smoked throughout their middle years were one-third more likely to have memory loss or other mental impairment than men who had never smoked. Men who had smoked at one time but quit also had some memory loss, but not as much as the continuous smokers.

If you haven't kicked the habit, now might be the time, before you lose any more of your precious memories.

Revitalize with B vitamins. Vitamins are vital to good health, and B vitamins are particularly vital to your brain's health. B vitamins work together, but a few are especially important if you want to keep your memory sharp.

- **Vitamin B12 (cobalamin).** If you don't get enough B12, you could develop pernicious anemia, which causes symptoms like pale skin, fatigue, and weakness. However, long before you show any other signs of low B12 levels, you could suffer memory loss. One study found that among people with pernicious anemia, 71 percent also had short-term memory loss. Treatment with B12 restored memory in most of them in less than a month. One reason B12 is important to brain health is that it helps your body manufacture neurotransmitters, chemicals that help carry messages between nerves and your brain. If you are a vegetarian, you may need to take supplements, since B12 is only found in foods from animals. The RDA for B12 is 2.4 mcg for people age 14 and older, but some memory experts recommend 100, even 1,000 mcg daily. Good food sources for vitamin B12 include red meat, salmon, and dairy products.

- **Vitamin B1 (thiamin).** This vitamin helps nerve signals travel from your brain to different parts of your body. A severe deficiency of thiamin can lead to beriberi, a disease that can cause mental disturbances. If you drink a lot of alcohol, you should be particularly careful to get plenty of B1. Alcohol decreases the absorption of thiamin in the intestines and increases the loss of thiamin in your urine. This can lead to a condition called Korsakoff's psychosis, which causes severe amnesia. Without prompt treatment of intravenous thiamin, this condition may be irreversible, resulting in permanent, disabling memory loss. The RDA for thiamin is 1.2 mg for adult males, and 1.1 mg for adult females. Good food sources of thiamin include wheat germ, nuts, beans, and rice.

- **Folic acid.** If you don't get enough folic acid in your diet, you could suffer mental and emotional problems, including depression and schizophrenia. The RDA for folic acid is 400 mcg for adult men and women. Good food sources include most plant foods, especially beans and green leafy vegetables.

Conditions that sabotage your memory

Everyone knows that Alzheimer's disease causes memory loss. But you may not know that other conditions also can sabotage your memory. If you have one of these illnesses, take heart. Memory loss is one symptom you may be able to reverse.

Depression. The most obvious symptom of depression may be simply feeling sad. However, people with depression may also have other symptoms, including forgetfulness.

Chronic fatigue syndrome. If you're tired all the time no matter how much rest you get, you may have this disease. Other symptoms include forgetfulness, joint or muscle pain, weakness, and mood swings.

Lupus. Systemic lupus erythematosus can inflame your brain's blood vessels, leading to memory loss. Other symptoms include weight and hair loss, fatigue, arthritis, and a facial rash. Drug treatment may correct memory problems associated with this disease.

Lyme disease. A tick bite may set off this disease that can cause joint pain, fever and chills, and memory and speech difficulties. Antibiotic treatment should reverse these problems.

Head injury. Sometimes a head injury that seems minor can cause mental problems that develop weeks or even months afterward.

Hypothyroidism. An underactive thyroid gland may cause you to be forgetful, tired, and depressed. Other symptoms include dry, yellowish skin, hoarse voice, and hair loss. This condition is easily controlled with synthetic hormones.

Vitamin deficiency. A deficiency of B vitamins may cause memory loss and other mental disturbances.

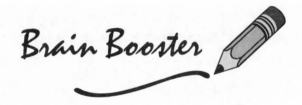

Memory checkup

Answer these questions to see how your memory for everyday things compares with others. Give yourself a score of 1 to 9 for each of the questions, then add up your scores. Use the following guide for scoring.

Not at all in the last six months **1 point**	About once a month **4 points**	More than once a week but less than once a day **7 points**
About once in the last six months **2 points**	More than once a month but less than once a week **5 points**	About once a day **8 points**
More than once in the last six months but less than once a month **3 points**	About once a week **6 points**	More than once a day **9 points**

1. Do you forget where you have put things? Lose things around the house?
2. Do you fail to recognize places that you are told you have often been to before?
3. Do you find television stories difficult to follow?
4. Have you forgotten a change in your daily routine, such as a change in the place where something is kept, or a change in the time something happens? Have you followed your old routine by mistake?
5. Have you had to go back to check whether you have done something that you meant to do?
6. Have you forgotten when something happened? For example, whether something happened yesterday or last week?
7. Have you completely forgotten to take things with you, or left things behind and had to go back and fetch them?
8. Have you forgotten that you were told something yesterday or a few days ago, and had to be reminded about it?
9. Have you started to read something (a book or a newspaper/magazine article) without realizing you have read it before?
10. Have you let yourself ramble on about unimportant or irrelevant things?

11. Have you failed to recognize, by sight, close relatives or friends that you meet frequently?

12. Have you had difficulty picking up a new skill? For example, learning a new game or operating a new gadget after you have practiced once or twice?

13. Have you found that a word is "on the tip of your tongue?" You know what it is but cannot quite find it.

14. Have you completely forgotten to do things you said you would do, and things you planned to do?

15. Have you forgotten important details of what you did or what happened to you the day before?

16. When talking to someone, have you forgotten what you have just said? Maybe saying "What was I talking about?" or "Where was I?"

17. When reading a newspaper or magazine, have you been unable to follow the thread of a story or lost track of what it is about?

18. Have you forgotten to tell somebody something important? Forgotten to pass on a message or remind someone of something?

19. Have you forgotten important details about yourself? For example, your date of birth or where you live?

20. Have you gotten the details of what someone had told you mixed up and confused?

21. Have you told someone a story or joke that you have told them already?

22. Have you forgotten details of things you do regularly, whether at home or at work? For example, details of what to do, or at what time to do something?

23. Have you found that the faces of famous people, seen on television or in photographs, look unfamiliar?

24. Have you forgotten where things are normally kept or looked for them in the wrong place?

25. (a) Have you gotten lost or taken a wrong turn on a journey, a walk, or in a building where you have OFTEN been before?
    (b) Have you gotten lost or taken a wrong turn on a journey, a walk, or in a building where you have only been ONCE OR TWICE before?

26. Have you done some routine thing twice by mistake? For example, putting two bags of tea in the teapot, or going to brush/comb your hair when you have just done so?

27. Have you repeated to someone what you have just told them or asked them the same question twice?

Your Memory: A User's Guide, Alan Baddeley, Prion Books, Ltd.

When you've tallied your score, turn to the *Solutions to Brain boosters and teasers* section at the back of the book to find out what it means.

Sharper thinking

Simple ways to boost your brain power

Thinking sounds like about the most natural thing in the world, and it is. But there are many kinds of thinking. For instance, the almost automatic thinking that reminds your fingers how to tie your shoes is very different from the focused, challenging thinking that goes into, say, piecing together the clues in a murder mystery. Because thinking in general is considered so natural, logical thinking is also considered natural. This is simply not true.

In order to think clearly and make logical decisions, we have to know what steps go into the process. Like any other weapon or tool, a brain is much more powerful in the hands of someone who knows how to get the best use out of it.

Are your thinking skills up to par? A little rusty, perhaps?

Turning that around might be a simple matter of re-learning the basics of sharp, logical thought. This chapter will examine the processes that allow you to use your mind to your best advantage.

If you sometimes feel like the edge of your thinking tool has been blunted and nicked from misuse, read on. We'll have that bean sharpened up in no time!

8 steps to foolproof decision making

Let's face it. Sometimes it's hard to make decisions, especially important ones. You go back and forth, agonize over your choices, and in the end, you may not do anything at all. Sound familiar? Well, you're not alone. Many of us have problems making decisions because we're so caught up in doing the "right" thing.

What you need to do is cut through the haze and get a clear picture of your situation. Whether you're picking a restaurant for dinner or a doctor to perform heart surgery, you can do it easily by following these eight simple steps.

Gather all related information. Try to find out as much about the situation as you possibly can, and then be open to new information later on. After looking at the situation from all angles, ask yourself (and perhaps others) why the situation stands as it does. In coming to a good decision, it is often the "why" that is more important than the "what."

Have confidence. Be confident that you will make the right decision. Don't sabotage yourself with needless fears or concerns. Instead, march on with confidence and faith in your decision-making ability.

Remain calm. Most decisions in life involve and affect ourselves and the people close to us. Of course, that makes it difficult to remain cool, calm, and collected when making major decisions. But that's exactly what you must do. If you become emotional, you won't be able to see the situation clearly. Then you can't make a fair, objective decision.

Be skeptical. Most of us are willing to believe what we hear, particularly when it comes from someone we love. If you want to make a good decision, pretend you're a judge in an important trial and listen with a neutral, impartial ear.

Consider all possible options. You may want to grab the obvious solution, especially when you're in a hurry. Don't do it! Take the time to consider other possibilities and solutions. How about a little brainstorming? Some of the best ideas have come out of this type of session.

Brainstorming works so well because you just throw out any and all ideas that come to mind. You may hear some odd ones, but don't tune them out immediately. A suggestion that sounds strange at first might just be what you're looking for if you keep an open mind.

Get a second opinion. Two heads are better than one, right? What better way to test an idea than to tell it to a friend? Try to find a friend who is not directly involved in the problem you are trying to solve. It should also be someone whose opinion and judgment you respect.

Try living your choice. If there's any way to try your idea first, by all means, do it. Even if this is not possible, just imagining yourself carrying out your decision step by step may be enough to make you see possible flaws.

Try killing your choice. If you're still happy with your choice, take the trial one step further. Examine every part of your solution carefully, searching for problems that could spring up. Don't feel bad if this step proves the solution is a bad one. Remember, your goal is to arrive at the best decision you can, not to settle for the first thing that springs into your head.

Sidestep 10 common pitfalls

Every decision you face is a small mystery that waits to be solved. You're the detective, and it's up to you to find all the clues. Along the way, there are plenty of mistakes to throw you off. Below are 10 common problems you must watch out for during your search for the right answer.

Identity crisis. A good rule is: First things first. When you set out, remember that before anything else, you need the facts. Your first step is always to size up the situation, and clearly identify the problem. Once you have all the facts and know what needs fixing, then you can move on to looking for your solution.

Prejudice. We all have our own likes and dislikes. When trying to solve a problem, however, these personal opinions can get in the way. You need to fight your own biases so you can see the situation as it truly is. To make a good decision, you must be able to think about a situation without reacting to it personally.

Extremes. Sometimes, things that look exactly the same are very different in small ways. For example, the harmless king snake often boasts red, yellow, and black rings of color on his skin. The coral snake has the same color rings in a slightly different order and is often mistaken for the king. The small detail is an important one, however — the coral snake's bite can kill a man. In cases like this, looking closely and carefully enough to get the full picture can be a matter of life and death.

The same is true for things that seem to be complete opposites. Quite often, two extremes share a lot of middle ground. So you need to be able to view things — facts, circumstances, people — in many different lights. Don't think black and white — think shades of gray. Most times, neither extreme is 100 percent right. The in-between gray area is usually where you'll find the truth.

Short-sightedness. Sometimes we are so wrapped up in finding an answer for today that we don't think about how this answer will work in the long term. A temporary solution is better than none at all, but you should try to do better than that. Always think about how your solution will work in future situations, then see if it still looks as good.

Carelessness. We all act a little lazy now and then. It can be quite tempting to just take a short look at a problem and form a quick decision based on this. But don't give in to the easy way out. Be complete in your search for facts, and take your time. The best decisions are those that are well thought out.

Poor judgment. Just as bad as the mistake of ignoring evidence is the problem of not understanding it. As Burton Hillis says, you have to distinguish between good, sound reasons and reasons that sound good. For example, you can say that lions and tigers are related because they both have fangs and feed on small mammals. Sounds good, but can't the same thing be said about bears? And wolves? And even snakes?

The better reason is that lions and tigers are related because their bodies have enough things in common to both be classified in the mammalian family *Felidea*.

The difference between a good argument and a worthless one is often rather slight. Your ability to see that difference and separate the two is what will determine your ability to come to good decisions.

Heart strings. "Follow your heart" is a popular saying, but it's not always the best advice. Really important decisions should involve your head. If you let your emotions rule your judgment, you may end up with solutions that you have not thought through properly. Let your head and your heart work together, and you'll usually make your best decisions.

Fatigue. Ever heard someone complain, "I'm so tired I can't think straight"? Well, it's not just an expression. Not getting enough sleep will wear you down, and not just physically. When you are tired, it is more difficult to think clearly, remember things, and make good decisions.

The pressure that often comes with a momentous decision can also wear on you, making the problem worse. Don't let it. Keep yourself focused on the problem, get enough sleep, and don't put too much pressure on yourself. When you're rested, your mind works more quickly and your attitude improves, and you're more prepared to make a good decision.

Inaction. Old Ben knew that most people's answer to a difficult challenge is to put it off as long as possible. But small problems have a way of becoming bigger ones when they are not dealt with quickly. Don't let decisions become harder because of laziness, delay, or fear. And don't try to fool yourself that simply worrying over a problem is a form of decision making. The best idea is to face the problem, make your decision, and then act upon that decision as soon as you can.

Early retirement. While we all would like to be perfect, sometimes we still make mistakes, bad choices, and bad decisions. When that happens, it's time to reevaluate. Go back to square one, and start the process all over again.

Unfortunately, very often we fall in love with our decisions and fail to recognize when they are not turning out the way we'd hoped. You should always be willing — and ready — to admit you've been wrong. That way, you can correct a bad decision before it makes matters even worse.

Putting your skills to work: Friday

Ready for a challenge? Test your new skills on this old favorite. If you get stumped, walk yourself through the problem using the decision-making techniques in this chapter:

A man rode into town on Friday. He stayed for three nights and then left on Friday. How could he do this?

Used with permission of Sterling Publishing Co., Inc., 387 Park Ave. S., New York, NY 10016 from *LATERAL THINKING PUZZLERS* by Paul Sloane, © 1991 by Paul Sloane

Check your answer in the *Solutions to Brain boosters and teasers* section at the back of the book.

Add up a solid solution

As you search for the one perfect solution, how do you keep your options straight in your head? Experts recommend taking notes to keep yourself on the right track. One good method for doing this is the PMI system.

PMI stands for plus, minus, and interesting. Begin by making three columns on a sheet of paper. Label the columns Plus, Minus, and Interesting. For the next few minutes, write down everything you can remember about your question or decision in the appropriate column.

When you feel like you've written down most of your thoughts, check the columns. Give yourself one point for each plus and minus in each column. If the pluses add up to more than the minuses, it's probably a good decision.

As a simple example, let's say you want to go out to dinner. You know of several good restaurants in town, but you've also heard some good things about a new restaurant where you've never eaten before. What do you do? How do you choose? If you decided to try the PMI technique, the beginning of your list might look something like this.

Plus	Minus	Interesting
Good reputation	No knowledge	New, unknown
Near home	Expensive	Fascinating building

When you're dealing with many different options, the differences between your idea can become hard to remember. Just seeing your thoughts in black and white often is enough to put choices back into perspective for you.

7 secrets of problem solving

Problem solving sounds a lot more complicated than decision making, but it isn't. Basically, if you know how to make good, sound decisions, you've got all the tools you need to create good, sound solutions to most of life's sticky problems. It's simply a matter of applying principles you already know. Follow these seven steps, and you'll be on your way to a more problem-free life.

Identify your problem. To do this, you need to look at the big picture. Sometimes people think a symptom of a problem is the problem itself. For example, you may fight with your husband over the way he spends money. But the real problem may be your fear that he'll lose his job during the company reorganization. Recognizing and dealing with the main problem at this step can save you many big headaches down the road.

Make a list of all possible solutions. Once you know what the problem is, the next step is to come up with a solution. This is a good time to sit back, relax, and let your imagination go wild. Try to think of a thousand different solutions; jot down everything from the practical and obvious to the fantastic and humorous.

This type of idea session is called brainstorming, and it works best when you do it with others. Find friends to help you who are bright and want to help. Make sure you get as many ideas out in the open as possible. You never know if the best answer is hiding just around the next corner. For more tips on fun and effective brainstorming techniques, see "Brainstorming: The path to creative solutions," beginning on page 85.

Evaluate and narrow your choices. When you've got a lot of possible solutions on the table, it's time to compare them to each other. Pick them apart, try to figure how they might fail or why one may be stronger than the others. Toss out any that probably won't work, and begin to focus on your strongest. Talk to others who have faced this problem in the past, if possible. Learn from their mistakes and their successes.

Choose the solution that seems best. Once you've narrowed down your choices, pick the one that seems best, and go with it. This is not to say you should make your final decision lightly. But you should make it quickly enough for the solution to work.

Try the solution you choose. Give it a go! Once you've made your selection and gotten your solution off the ground, get behind it 100 percent. Don't be half-hearted about it. If the decision was good enough to choose, it deserves a fair shake. Follow your plan closely, and don't second-guess yourself. Even if your solution fails, you won't know why unless you work it through to the end.

Evaluate your choice. Here's where the hard work comes in. Once you've seen how your solution works, you should step back and rate your performance. This is important even if you think you've done a fantastic job. It will give you a better picture of why your solution succeeded, or, perhaps more importantly, why it failed. Only by studying and acknowledging your mistakes will you be able to avoid them in the future.

Repeat the last two steps. Do it until you've found the best solution. Don't be afraid to try, try again. Rarely does any new thing succeed on the first attempt. Only by trying a number of different ways are you sure to come up with the best one. The bottom line is, don't get discouraged, and don't quit. This is the only way to succeed.

If you need inspiration, take a look at Thomas Edison. Despite being perhaps history's most inspired inventor, his light bulb project failed hundreds upon hundreds of times before it finally succeeded. As proof of his effective problem-solving techniques, Edison's long-burning light bulb remains almost unchanged in design to this day.

Putting your skills to work:
The coal, carrot, and scarf

This puzzle's a little harder. Remember, like most problems in life, this one has a logical solution — it's just not standing right out in the open. Take your time, follow the problem-solving steps you've learned, and be willing to look at the question from several different perspectives. Have fun!

Five pieces of coal, a carrot, and a scarf are lying on the lawn. Nobody put them on the lawn, but there is a perfectly logical reason why they should be there. What is it?

Used with permission of Sterling Publishing Co., Inc., 387 Park Ave. S., New York, NY 10016 from *LATERAL THINKING PUZZLERS* by Paul Sloane, © 1991 by Paul Sloane

Check your answer in the *Solutions to Brain boosters and teasers* section at the back of the book.

Brainstorming: The path to creative solutions

Brainstorming is a very important part of problem solving as well as a powerful tool. A lot of great solutions come right out of brainstorming sessions because it sparks your creativity and encourages you to think in new ways. If you've never tried brainstorming, it might seem a little awkward at first. Here are some tips to get your brainstorming sessions off to a good start:

Find a friend. Although it's perfectly fine to brainstorm alone, it works best when you put two or more heads together. More heads produce more thoughts and opinions and perspectives, and that means more ideas.

Use a pen. It is important to write down the ideas as they come to you. Don't make the mistake of thinking you can just remember the good ones or that you'll just brainstorm until you come up with a good idea. A big part of brainstorming is sticking to it, kicking around ideas until you've got nothing left. You'll need those notes later.

Let yourself go. The point of brainstorming is to get out new ideas and lots of them. As soon as you think of one, jot it down and move on. Don't think about your idea, judge it, or try to develop it, not yet. For now, concentrate on getting as many ideas as possible, not worrying whether the ones you come up with are good or bad.

Listen to repetition. If an idea is suggested twice, write it down twice. Chances are, the two ideas are not exactly the same, and one version might have the slight difference that makes the idea a workable one.

Laugh a little. Don't be afraid to write down unusual or even goofy ideas. Often new ideas seem silly just because they've never been tried before. It could be that a fresh, innovative solution is hiding somewhere in your sense of humor.

Keep the problem in sight. Through it all, keep the problem you are trying to solve clear in your mind. If done well, brainstorming can be a lot of fun, which means you can easily stray away from the question at hand. That's fine, but be sure to remind yourself and the group that your overall goal is solving that problem.

Procrastination: Winning the delay relay

To be a good problem solver, you must be willing to take on the tasks and challenges that face you. Perhaps nothing gets in the way of personal progress and good decisions more than constant delay.

Why do we put off things that need to get done? Probably because many of us — perhaps most of us — are born with a strong tendency to procrastinate. We have many excuses: we're tired, we don't want to face a difficult situation, we're genuinely lazy. There are as many reasons as there are procrastinators.

The trouble with procrastination is that although it seems harmless enough, it is an addictive habit. It leads to many unfortunate ends such as guilt, self-doubt, anxiety, and a general feeling that you have lost control and are powerless in your life. Depression is just around the next corner, because when you are not moving forward in life, you are either standing still or losing ground. And neither of these makes you feel good about yourself.

The usual justification for procrastinating is the notion that, if you wait long enough, your problems will go away by themselves. Of course this sounds silly in the clear light of day, but when your mind decides to work on you, its arguments can be pretty convincing.

Procrastination is a battle, but one you can win. To do this, you must convince yourself that you can make a difference in your own life. Start by focusing on the three basic elements of your problem.

Action changes. These are some of the actual, physical steps that will help you get moving. Remember, do not delay — put one of these valuable techniques into practice today.

- **Start small.** Take small steps at first. Don't try to do too much or win back all the time you've ever lost at once. Plan just a few steps at a time, but take those steps.

- **Write down your goals.** Design clear goals for yourself and write them down. Make them specific and attainable, things that you can reasonably accomplish. Writing down your goals reinforces them and keeps them fresh in your mind. This approach also gives you the satisfaction of physically crossing off each goal after you've accomplished it.

- **Keep goal lists updated.** Keeping lists up-to-date will help you stay on top of the many demands on your time. Review your goals regularly to see how well you are doing. You should have separate lists for things you need to keep ahead of (such as bills), things you have to catch up on (like filing receipts), and things to move forward on (call for those summer vacation brochures).

- **Turn the tables.** Use the activities you usually procrastinate with as rewards for not putting things off. For example: "I won't let myself do the crossword puzzle until I've cleaned out the bathtub." By rewarding yourself this way, you can turn a traditional roadblock into part of your accomplishment.

- **Be flexible.** Keep an open mind, and always have room on your plate for new things that could pop up. If you are too rigid in your schedule, you will not be able to adapt to changes or surprises. So stay loose, and be ready to deal with new items as they arise.

Mental changes. All the physical tricks in the world won't help you if you don't win the battle of the mind. It is your mind that devises the excuses and justification schemes that fuel procrastination. But a mind that can work against you in this way can certainly be trained to work for you. The following tips will help keep your head in the game.

- **Name your goal.** If you acknowledge the goal of overcoming procrastination, you place it directly in front of you and face it down every day. Commit yourself to this goal, and keep it in mind whenever you find yourself returning to old habits.

- **Be on your guard.** Be ready to recognize the ploys of procrastination. Your mind has convinced you before that delay was okay, and it will probably try again. Keep a mental list of the situations when it was easiest for you to slip into procrastination, and prepare yourself to be strong when those situations come around.

- **Conquer the "tomorrow syndrome."** This is the most common of all mental tricks. Our mind tells us, very simply, that if it has waited this long, it can surely wait one more day. And surely it will be easier to do tomorrow! Don't believe it. You can play that game day after day for years.

- **Beware of "double-tomorrow."** This is the slightly sneakier cousin of the tomorrow syndrome, and you need to face it, too. It's when you tell yourself you'll do something just as soon as some other "prerequisite" falls into place. Your mind tries to make you believe that your ability to act depends on things that are beyond your control. This is rarely the case. If you wait for everything to be perfect, you'll never start anything.

Emotional changes. Procrastination is an emotional issue because many of the tactics it uses play on our self-esteem, self-image, or security. But don't let procrastination intimidate you. Take charge of your mind and your emotions, and move forward.

- **Have a positive outlook.** Don't see tasks as ordeals. Instead, see them as challenges. Often, just looking at something as an adventure or an opportunity instead of as a chore or duty can make all the difference in your enthusiasm.

- **Go easy on yourself.** You should push yourself to succeed, but don't push too hard. Don't belittle yourself; inspire yourself. Reward yourself for victories and accomplishments, but don't beat yourself up over setbacks. There will be plenty of each along the way, so be prepared.

- **Relax.** Many people put things off because of various forms of anxiety, fear, pressure, and stress. Don't let this happen to you. Realize that tension and nervousness are natural parts of life, and you can fight through them. Take time to do the things that relax you, whether it is meditation, rest, exercise, or a simple game of checkers. Staying on an even keel in general will keep you afloat when storms of stress blow up.

The 5-minute jump-start

For many people, the first step is the hardest step. If this is true for you, try this exercise to get yourself going. Dedicate just five minutes to a task, and during those five minutes, get as much done on it as you can. When your time is up, decide if you want to go another five minutes, then do.

Repeat these five-minute cycles as many times in a row as you want. When you decide to stop, if you have not yet completed your project, take a final five minutes to plan out where you will pick up when you come back to finish.

Fight falsehood with good old-fashioned logic

For a lot of us, "logic" is a scary word. To many people, it sounds like some sort of mental game that brainiacs play in university laboratories. But it's really not scary at all. It is something we use every day, only some people use it better than others.

Logic is nothing more than the ability to figure out whether or not the reasons for a statement really make that statement true. If the reasons are good ones, the statement is logical. That's all there is to it. When you can tell between good reasons and bad ones, you are using logic. And when you combine a firm grasp of logic with solid decision making skills, you're using the power of critical thinking.

Logic and critical thinking are powerful tools that anyone can master. Your mind already has the skills it needs, but it also contains the pitfalls that can throw logic out the window at a moment's notice. Learning to guard against these errors is what critical thinking is all about.

The lazy mind. If you want to think logically, the best way to do it is to keep reminding yourself of what makes a logical statement. Many people get confused not because they're unintelligent but because they don't listen with self-discipline. Lazy thinkers tend to accept whatever "sounds good," as opposed to what really makes the most sense.

This is not to say that you must always be on your toes, constantly applying rules of logic and watching out for mistakes. Far from it. Once you know the few simple traps that give people the most problems, it will become second nature to keep them in mind, and critical thinking will become a snap.

The danger of false assumptions. We all make assumptions every day. You may assume that your husband will take out the garbage on trash day or that your wife will pick up your suit at the drycleaners. Or you may write out a check assuming there is enough money in your bank account to cover your purchase.

When we assume, we accept something as true without any actual proof. Of course, we have to do this in our day-to-day life. If we had to prove everything all the time, we'd never leave the house. But when you are counting on your critical thinking to help you make the right choice, assumptions are your number one no-no.

Resist the urge to assume. Demand proof, even when you are pretty sure something is true. If you naturally tend to favor one side, do most of your looking for facts that prove the opposite. Make yourself objective by pushing aside your assumptions.

A good way to guard against your natural preferences is to think about what assumptions you are likely to make. Your biases and beliefs are hard to fight, but you need to keep them in check. Keeping them in mind as you approach a situation will help you steer clear of assumptions based on your expectations and think your way clear to the logical conclusion.

The impulsive mind. If you've ever tried brainstorming, you know that blurting out the first idea that comes to your mind is useful for sparking creativity and getting lots of ideas. Or in a casual conversation, you might answer a question by saying, "Well, just off the top of my head..." This is all fine for talk among friends, but not if you're trying to find a logical solution.

Your first thought is usually an instinct reaction, based not on fact but on prejudice, personal tastes, or other things you already know. Therefore, it is probably an assumption, since it hasn't been proven.

Another part of your body that you should doubt is your "gut." Many people have great faith in their instincts, in their "gut reactions," but such responses have no place in the world of logic. What you need isn't in your gut or your heart but in your head.

So take your time with your decision. Learning to trust logic over your instinct is a sure sign of the seasoned critical thinker.

Being misled by others. Being misled doesn't necessarily mean being lied to, but the result is the same. People mislead each other a thousand times a day, in a thousand different ways and for a thousand different reasons. Seems like a lot to look out for, doesn't it? Well, it is and it isn't. The easiest way is to always remember what makes a statement logical, and to always remember to look for that.

One big reason people abandon their logic is out of loyalty. When our friends make statements, we tend to believe them. Our friendship is a form of prejudice. It's not nice to think that our friends might lie to us, but for the sake of logic, this possibility should always be considered. Proof is needed to back up any statement no matter who makes it.

Advertisers use this loyalty to sell all sorts of products. They pay athletes and movie actors a lot of money to go on TV and tell people to buy fancy shoes and cars. Fans of these stars respond because they like the celebrities and want to believe them. They don't think about the fact that playing football or acting in movies doesn't make someone an expert on these products, or even necessarily honest. But that's what we should be looking for — proof, not packaging.

When making decisions, pay attention to the message and the facts. Think about the messenger as well as your feelings for him. If you have feelings for the messenger — good feelings or bad — remember that these feelings could get in the way of your logic.

Messengers also have many motivations, and you should remember these too. It's nice to think that everyone has your best interest at heart, but this just isn't so. Be on the lookout for such "tricks" as flattery and humor. Someone who compliments your hair or makes you laugh, such as a salesman might, is more likely to make you believe him. Remember, compliments and laughs and even friendship are never reasons to believe anybody.

The lure of false associations. A is like B, and B is like C. Therefore, A is like C. Right? Wrong. Or rather, not necessarily. This is the classic example of lazy man's logic. It is what is known as a faulty association.

Here is another example: Joe drank a glass of water at 3 o'clock. Joe also got a headache at 3 o'clock. Therefore, drinking a glass of water gave Joe a headache.

What's wrong with this reasoning? The mistake is that even though the conclusion may be true, it is not necessarily true. True, Joe got a headache at the same time he drank a glass of water. However, a rock also could have fallen on Joe's head at 3 o'clock, and that could have caused the headache.

When dealing with logic, you have to look for only what is necessarily true. Don't assume two items or events are related just because they look the same or because they happened at the same time.

When two things seem to be the same, that's when you have to look closely to find their differences. Often, the subtle differences between two similar things can give away the fact that they are not related to each other.

Putting your skills to work:
The man in the bar

Think you've got problem solving mastered? This one's a real noodle scratcher. Solve this problem, and you're qualified as an officially logical thinker.

A man walks into a bar and asks the barman for a glass of water. The barman pulls out a gun and points it at the man. The man says 'Thank you' and walks out. Why?

Used with permission of Sterling Publishing Co., Inc., 387 Park Ave. S., New York, NY 10016 from *LATERAL THINKING PUZZLERS* by Paul Sloane, © 1991 by Paul Sloane

Check your answer in the *Solutions to Brain boosters and teasers* section at the back of the book.

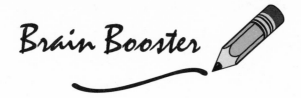

Test your powers of observation and memory

One of the keys to better thinking is keen observation — seeing what is actually in front of your eyes, instead of what you expect to see. Another is remembering what you have observed. See how well these skills work together for you.

Before you read these questions, turn to the end of the *Solutions to Brain boosters and teasers* section at the back of the book and look at the picture for 30 seconds. Then turn back here and take the test.

1. Was the mother wearing a dress, a skirt and blouse, or pants and a top?

2. Which hand was she using to brush the girl's hair?

3. Where was the mother's other hand?

4. Was the mother a blond or a brunette?

5. Was the child's hair the same color as the mother's hair?

6. Who in the picture was wearing shoes — the mother, the child, or both mother and child?

7. Was the child holding a stuffed bear, a doll, or a book?

8. Was it the child's face, the mother's face, or the child's hair that was reflected in the mirror?

9. Was the child sitting in a chair, standing beside a chair, or kneeling on the floor?

10. Name two of the three objects on the dresser.

Check your answers in the *Solutions to Brain boosters and teasers* section at the back of the book.

Creativity

Awaken your imagination

At Zoo Atlanta, you can buy paintings created by Starlet the elephant, usually something with bold red strokes appropriate for a creature named after Scarlett O'Hara. Does this mean Starlet has a creative mind? Actually, she's probably pretty unaware of what she's putting on the canvas with the paintbrush curled up in her trunk. Scientists call creativity "species specific," which means it is a trait possessed only by humans.

The human mind is not only capable of being creative, it may need to be creative. Studies find that people who score high on tests of creativity also tend to have high levels of self-confidence and low levels of anxiety. Becoming a more creative person may make you a happier, more confident person.

If you were asked to make a list of creative people, you might list names like Da Vinci, Edison, Shakespeare, Van Gogh, or Edgar Allen Poe. These people were all certainly creative, and even considered geniuses. But if you want to see a creative person up close and personal, take a look in the mirror.

You don't have to paint a masterpiece or write a best selling novel or invent a time machine to be creative. All you need is your own imagination. Every time you try a new ingredient in a recipe or rearrange your furniture, you are exercising your creativity.

Everyone has the ability to be creative. It's all a matter of expression. How do you express your creative side? Do you like to needlework, knit, or quilt? Do you write interesting letters to your friends? Do you plant colorful flowers in your yard, or build model airplanes?

Creativity can improve your mind and your life. Discover how to awaken the creative person inside you.

Get your creative juices flowing

You think of yourself as a humdrum kind of person without a creative bone in your body. You have beige furniture in your house, with white walls and not a sign of artwork or needlework anywhere. But you long to be considered imaginative and talented. Can you make yourself more creative?

Although creativity may come more easily to some people, everyone has that ability. It's just a matter of letting those creative juices flow.

Think creative. First of all, stop thinking of yourself as humdrum. "As a man thinketh, so is he." In other words, you are what you think. Consider yourself interesting and creative, and you will convince yourself and everyone else that you are.

Write it down. You don't have to be a Hemingway to express yourself on paper. Keep a daily journal of your most interesting thoughts and ideas. Don't worry about style or grammar. Just jot down quickly whatever's in your mind — how you feel, what you observed during the day, your opinion of a news story. Go back over your journals periodically and see how much you've changed.

Open your mind. A closed mind gathers no new ideas. To be creative, you must be ready and willing to say, "Why not?" The instant camera was invented because Edward Land's young daughter asked him why they had to wait to see the pictures they were taking while vacationing. Instead of saying, "Just because that's the way it works," Edward said, "Good question." He set to work on the problem, and the instant Polaroid camera made its appearance soon afterward.

Vary your interests. You probably have a few things you are interested in, but if you cultivate interest in a wide variety of subjects, you will give your mind and your imagination a broader base for ideas. If you normally only read the sports section of the newspaper, add the world news. If you usually read science fiction, try a historical romance.

Kick back. If you're too busy to take a breath, you're too busy to be creative. Slow down. Give yourself time to relax, and just let your thoughts wander. Philo Farnsworth came up with the idea for television while sitting on a hillside looking at some fields. The lines in the fields gave him the inspiration for creating pictures made of rows of light and dark dots. If he had been too busy to relax and observe, you might not be able to watch your favorite shows today.

Laugh more. A sense of humor can be a tool for creativity. In one study, people who watched a short comedy film of television bloopers did better on a test requiring creative solutions that people who exercised or watched a film about math. Be playful. Use different colored pens, draw ideas instead of writing them down, etc.

Take a different tack. In sailing, when the wind dies in one direction, you change your tack to take advantage of a different wind current. Thinking creatively requires the same tactics. If what you're doing isn't working, try something different, because if you always do what you've always done, you'll always get what you've always gotten.

Let the ideas flow. A great way to generate creative ideas is to brainstorm with your friends or co-workers. (See the *Sharper thinking* chapter for tips on brainstorming.) However, if you're shy, or if you just don't have other people handy to help, you can try brainwriting. Just grab a pen and paper and jot down whatever pops into your head, no matter how silly. The silliest ideas sometimes lead you to the most brilliant ones.

Ask open-ended questions. Whenever you're faced with a problem that requires a creative solution, try asking yourself questions about the situation that can't be answered with a simple yes or no. For example, instead of asking "Will I get a raise soon?" ask, "What are some things I can do to make my boss think I deserve a raise?"

Observe closely. Try this experiment of your observational powers. Write down names of colors on a piece of paper using markers in different colors from the word. For example, write the word red with a green marker, the word black with a yellow marker, etc. Then quickly try to name the color of the ink used to print each word. You might be surprised at how difficult it is! This is because the left side of your brain sees the word while your "right brain" sees the color. Become an up-close and personal observer and see what is actually there — not what you expect to see.

Play creative games. Put your imagination to work with some friends. The next time you have a get-together, play some creative games. A game of charades forces you to come up with creative ways to express yourself without words. Pictionary does the same thing, but it arms you with paper and pencil so you can draw out your thoughts.

Catch some zzz's. Too little sleep can sap your creative powers. When you're tired, you don't think as clearly, and your imagination suffers. Also, the dreams you have while you're sleeping can be a great inspiration. See the *Dreaming* chapter for help in tapping this source of creative power.

Have a creative space. Your environment can influence your creative powers. Many famous writers and artists fill their work area with objects that inspire them. Others prefer to work outdoors, letting nature provide inspiration. The best environments are usually ones that feed all your senses, filled with pleasant things to look at, listen to, smell, and touch. Find out what kind of surroundings encourage you to loosen up and let your imagination fly.

Everyday creativity

Give your creativity a workout with this simple exercise. Think of a common everyday object – for example, a brick, a toothpick, or a rubberband. Now, how many uses can you list for that object? It's OK to start with the obvious. A brick is a great building material. But how about using a brick as a paperweight or a doorstop? You get the idea. Have a friend join you in this exercise, and compare lists afterward.

Sidestep stumbling blocks to creativity

You're ready to become a more creative person. But watch out for blocks in your path to creativity that will cause you to remain in a rut.

Lessen stress. Sometimes you might work better under a deadline. The adrenaline starts to flow, and you put forth extra effort. After a while, however, the stress becomes counterproductive, and your mind goes on a sit-down strike. A relaxed state of mind is conducive to creativity. For help in controlling stress, see the tips in the *Mindpower* chapter.

No fear. Franklin Roosevelt said "The only thing we have to fear is fear itself." Fear of failure may be the greatest stumbling block to creativity. Don't be afraid to make mistakes — everyone makes mistakes. Without someone's willingness to take chances, inventions like the lightbulb and the airplane would not exist.

In fact, one of the most important inventions to modern teenagers, the telephone, was based on a mistake. Alexander Graham Bell reportedly was inspired to start work on the concept of the telephone after reading a report, written in German, which he thought described such an instrument. Later, he discovered that he had misunderstood the report, which described something else entirely.

Let go of logic. Logic holds an important place in the decision-making process. However, all logic and no play makes creativity go away. Sometimes what seems illogical can be a valid solution. Consider all possibilities no matter how silly they may seem.

Change your perspective. It's taken you years of living to develop your personality and your perspective. However, when a problem calls for a creative solution, try someone else's perspective on for size. Put yourself in another person's shoes. How would your Uncle Lou solve this problem? What would your wacky friend Dodie think about the situation? Sometimes seeing things through someone else's eyes can open up your own eyes to an obvious solution.

Lose control. Toss your need for power and control. Otherwise, you'll control your creativity right out the door. You don't have to be in charge of every situation. Sometimes it's better to just go with the flow.

Nix the negative. Nothing squashes creativity like a negative attitude. Put the critical part of your mind on hold. Try to eliminate "can't" and "don't" from your vocabulary for a while.

Don't rush. True creativity takes time. Don't be discouraged if you don't see immediate results. It took the Wright brothers five years of work to create their first airplane.

An enlightening way to creativity

Thomas Edison was someone who knew how to make the most of his creative instincts. He recognized that his best creative insights came when he was in the stage between alertness and sleep.

Knowing this, he devised a method to help himself not let any creative ideas slip away during sleep by sitting in a comfortable chair with his arms draped over the sides holding two heavy metal balls over two metal pans. He would let himself drift off toward sleep until he was awakened by the crash of the balls into the metal pans. It was at the point, he notes, that he had his best creative insights.

This method must have worked well for Edison, because by the end of his life, he held patents for more than 1,200 inventions.

7 super ways to get inspired

Creativity is a valuable skill in the business world. It seems that everywhere you turn, you find seminars designed to teach business people how to think creatively. Thanks in part to this interest, many techniques for creative thinking have been developed. You can use some of them to inspire you.

Think random thoughts. One of the most often-used techniques for inspiring creative solutions is the random input technique. Newton supposedly got the idea of gravity when he was hit on the head by an apple falling from a tree. Chance events like that can sometimes be the spark that ignites fresh thoughts.

Random input uses a chance event, or in this case, a word, to generate new ideas. You simply choose a word at random and then list all the associations and qualities of the word. You then see how each of the items on your list might apply to your current problem.

The words should be nouns, and there are several ways to choose them. You can open a dictionary, close your eyes, and point. You can write words on slips of paper, put them in a bag, and then draw one. You can cut out pictures of items, and choose one of them. You can even use the wonders of modern technology, and try a random-word computer program.

Put it in reverse. Sometimes opposites attract creative solutions. Problem reversal is a technique that uses opposites as inspiration. Try looking at your problem in reverse. Define what something is *not* or figure out what other people are *not* doing. For example, if you're trying to make the grass grow on your lawn, think about all the things you could do to keep it from growing.

Question it. The favorite word of most 4-year-olds is "why." That's because they are eager to learn how things work. You can use the same technique to jog your creativity. When you have a problem, ask yourself the six universal questions: who, what, when, where, why, and how. For example, why did it occur? How did it happen? What can you do about it? Who might be able to help you? Finally, where and when can you solve the problem?

Put on your thinking hats. Some of the world's largest companies use a method called the Six Thinking Hats invented by Dr. Edward DeBono. In this technique, each colored hat represents a direction for thinking.

- **White hat.** White represents facts and figures. You have to consider the facts when making any decision.

- **Red hat.** This hat covers intuition and emotions. Feelings and intuition can be valid points in creative solutions.

- **Black hat.** This hat is a caution signal. Although not necessarily negative, black covers why a suggestion may not be a wise one.

- **Yellow hat.** The logical yellow hat helps you look at why something might work and what benefits are offered in a particular idea.

- **Green hat.** This is the creative hat. It represents the interesting and unique ideas.

- **Blue hat**. The blue hat is the overseer. It looks not at the problem itself, but at how you are thinking about the problem.

When trying to come up with creative solutions to problems, put on one thinking hat at a time. Use each color to come up with imaginative and interesting ideas.

Follow a map. Mind mapping is a thinking technique created by Tony Buzan, a well-known creativity expert. You just start in the center of a page, and write down your main idea. Then around that central idea, you add key words and associations, connected like roads on a map.

Force the issue. Have fun generating ideas with forced analogies. This method involves comparing your problem with something that has little or nothing to do with the problem. For example, "Our relationship is like a tennis shoe because ..." or "My job is like an apple ..."

Think laterally. Another popular method of creative problem solving is lateral thinking. This involves looking at a problem laterally, or sideways, and seeing more than the obvious solutions.

For example, you wake up in the middle of the night to the sound of a dripping faucet. You can't go back to sleep because the sound is driving you crazy. You can't call a plumber in the middle of the night, and you don't know how to fix the leak yourself. At the moment, the problem isn't the leak itself, but the noise it is making, keeping you awake.

Thinking laterally, you could place a wash cloth in the bottom of the sink. The water won't make a noise hitting the soft cloth, and it will still allow the water to drain as the cloth becomes saturated.

*"It isn't that they can't see the solution.
It is that they can't see the problem."*

— G.K. Chesterson

Exercise 'jogs' your imagination

You're jogging along, thinking about nothing but putting one foot in front of the other and making it home without passing out. Suddenly, inspiration hits you from out of nowhere. You have a moment of great creativity without even trying.

What was responsible for this sudden inspiration? It could be your jogging shoes, or more likely, what you do in your jogging shoes.

Studies find that exercise enhances creativity. Many researchers think that exercise gives a boost to your creative side by giving your mood a boost. However, a recent study found that exercise improved creativity independent of mood.

People in the study took tests to assess their mood and creativity level after doing aerobic exercise for 25 minutes. Exercise increased positive mood as well as creativity. However, watching a video also increased positive mood but had no effect on creativity.

Exercise gets your blood flowing, delivering more oxygen to your brain. It also triggers the release of endorphins in your brain, which are responsible for the feeling of elation known as the "runner's high."

The rhythm of your exercise program can be a source of inspiration, too. The beat of footsteps, bicycle pedals, or swimming strokes can be soothing and meditative.

So, if you want to be more creative, go for a run and let your imagination run, too.

*"The creative person is both more primitive and more cultivated,
more destructive and more constructive,
a lot madder and a lot saner than the average person."*

— John V. Basmajian

Mood disorders: The dark side of creativity?

The image of a mad genius — hair standing on end with wild-looking eyes is a popular one. And interestingly, research finds that highly creative, artistic people may actually be more likely to suffer emotional disorders than most people. But don't let these seemingly grim facts dampen your quest for creativity. Being creative doesn't mean you will necessarily develop a mood disorder.

Arnold M. Ludwig, a psychiatrist at the University of Kentucky Medical Center, investigated the link between creative achievement and emotional turmoil.

He found that among prominent 20th-century poets, musical performers, and fiction writers, about three-fourths had serious psychological symptoms as adults. Between 46 to 77 percent of writers, poets, painters, and composers experienced serious depression. Manic depression, which affects less than 1 percent of the general population, afflicted 11 to 17 percent of prominent actors, poets, architects, and nonfiction writers.

This seems to support the link between mood disorders and artistic creativity. The question is: does one cause the other? Some researchers think so — others disagree.

Kay Redfield Jamison is one psychiatrist who believes highly creative people are more likely to suffer from depression and manic-depression. The author of the book *Touched with Fire: Manic-Depressive Illness and the Artistic Temperament* found that major

18th-century British poets were 20 times more likely to have been committed to a mental institution than the general public. They were also five times more likely to have committed suicide.

But, Jamison says, these extreme moods may have actually enhanced the artists' creativity and made their works even more powerful.

Does this mean you have to be manic-depressive to be a great artistic talent? Fortunately not. Developing an emotional disorder won't necessarily turn you into a creative genius. By the same token, being creative doesn't mean you are destined to develop a mental illness.

However, if you have a highly creative friend or loved one who seems to be irritable and depressed, or experiences wild mood swings, you may want to have their doctor check them out. Their moods may be due to more than just artistic eccentricity.

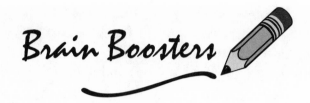

Candle-mounting problem

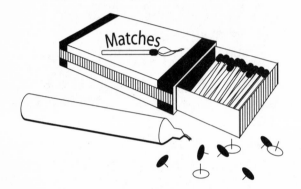

Using these materials, how would you mount the candle on a bulletin board?

Credit: Duncker, K. (1945). On problem solving. *Psychological Monographs,* 58 (Whole # 270)

Trivia quiz

1. What is the only 15-letter word that can be spelled without repeating a letter?

2. Which is the only state in the United States whose name has one syllable?

3. Is it true or false that if you go blind in one eye you'll lose half your vision?

4. Which has caused more human deaths, fleas or tigers?

5. Which meal do Americans skip most often?

6. Which sex is more likely to flash their lights to let oncoming drivers know about a traffic cop ahead?

7. Other than the fact that alligators don't shed crocodile tears, how can you tell these similar reptiles apart?

8. The man who invented the silencer — which makes a gun shot sound more like a "pop" than a "boom" — invented something else as well. Can you guess what?

9. Which requires more heating — to turn an ounce of snow to water or to bring an ounce of soup to a boil from room temperature?

10. Which is the only country in the world where you can see the sun rise on the Pacific Ocean and set on the Atlantic?

11. The Washington Cathedral has a stained glass window dedicated to scientists and technicians. What material in this window makes it unusual?

12. On which birthday can you most accurately calculate the height a child is likely to reach as an adult?

13. Which part of the body has the most brain space devoted to controlling it — the abdomen, the chest, or the thumb?

14. Which wood should you burn in your fireplace to get the most heat — ash, cherry, or poplar?

15. What happens to a goldfish's appearance if you put it in a stream of running water?

Check your answers in the *Solutions to Brain boosters and teasers* section at the back of the book.

Learning

It's never too late

You begin the learning process the day you are born. At its most basic, learning is nothing more than linking your senses to your memory. You sense something, notice how it affects you, and remember this information for future use.

In the first years of life, you learn at an incredible rate. Everything is new, interesting, and fascinating, and your memory soaks it all up. As you get older and grow familiar with the world, there are still millions of things to consider, try out, evaluate, and remember. The world is still your mind's playground.

And yet, it's easy to fall into the trap of ignoring this vast playground. Once you know the details of survival — when to eat, what work needs to be done, how to function as a member of a family — it's possible to click your brain onto auto-pilot. Television, which requires very little thought or actual attention, can get you into a rut that keeps your mind from getting any exercise.

Keeping your mind active is as important as exercising your body. The process and result of learning can help keep you mentally fit, guard against certain disorders, and make your life more fun and interesting. It might even help you live longer.

> *"Success is a state of mind. If you want success, start thinking of yourself as a success."*
>
> — Joyce Brothers

Enhance your learning style

You have your favorite ways of doing things, and learning is no exception. There are many different types of learning, but these are the four most common.

Visual learners. If you are a visual learner, you learn best using methods that have to do with sight. The most common example is reading, although it also includes other activities, such as looking at drawings, studying graphs and charts, and taking notes.

Verbal learners. Verbal learners are most successful when they learn through oral communication. Speaking out loud, conversing and exchanging ideas with others, talking to yourself, and repeating important facts are verbal methods of learning.

Auditory learners. This type is similar to the visual learner, except the natural preference lies in hearing instead of seeing. Auditory types learn best by listening to a lecture, an audio cassette, or music.

Kinesthetic learners. People who are kinesthetic learners don't learn well by studying books or listening to someone talk. They find learning easier by jumping in with both feet and physically "getting their hands on" the subject.

If you are a kinesthetic learner, you won't get much out of watching a video. On the other hand, a visual learner will get little out of a panel discussion. And here's why. If you are not comfortable or well-suited to the method of learning, your full attention will not be on the knowledge you are trying to absorb.

These labels are simply generalizations to help you figure out your natural preferences. Knowing your style can help you maximize your learning experience. You might learn well by using any combination of your senses, or all your senses at once.

Simple exercises sharpen your mind

Ruth Upchurch, who teaches kinesiology to both children and adults in the Atlanta area, believes everybody is a kinesthetic learner — up to a point.

She believes movement and physical activity are crucial to success in just about anything that involves your mind.

"Educational kinesiology is very important to the learning process, especially if someone has had problems in the development of their learning patterns," says Ms. Upchurch. "It can make anyone a better learner, young or old, even people with learning disabilities."

Ms. Upchurch teaches kinesiology sessions, also called "Edu-K" or "Brain Gym." This program instructs students on the use of specific body movements that can improve the way their minds work. As she explains it, your brain is divided into two halves, and each half has certain tasks it takes care of. In order to learn effectively, both halves have to be going full tilt at once, cooperating with each other and with the rest of your body. That's where Brain Gym comes in.

"Your learning patterns mirror the patterns of your development," Ms. Upchurch says. "Anything that interrupts those patterns, such as emotional trauma, injury, stress, or illness, can create a serious learning block. The Brain Gym program uses a series of 26 physical movements and a 5-step balancing process to integrate both sides of your brain and change those obstructed learning patterns. It does this by making that important connection between mind and body, getting every part of you on the same song sheet."

This type of program was originally designed for children with Attention Deficit Disorder and other learning problems. The goal was to calm the children and release their stored-up energy and stress so they could concentrate better in school. The techniques worked so well they were expanded for adults.

A series of simple physical exercises, like touching a left part of your body with your right hand or crossing your legs and arms at the same time, limbers the body and sharpens the mind.

"The point of the exercises is to get both halves of your brain working in unison and making the important connection between mind and body," says Ms. Upchurch. "Once everything is working from the same song sheet, you are balanced and clear and ready to learn faster and more completely than ever before."

Ms. Upchurch's younger students have seen remarkable results in improving their grades, reading ability, and organizational skills. And it's not just the kids, either. Brain Gym helps people of all ages overcome stumbling blocks in their learning. Problems with attention, motivation, creativity, and energy are just some of the difficulties Brain Gym has helped clear up.

Over the years, these principles have proven themselves so sound and the techniques so effective that today there is a full line of Edu-K systems. You can harness the power of kinesiology to improve anything from your study habits to your salesmanship to your golf game. For more information about these programs, contact the Educational Kinesiology Foundation at (800) 356-2109.

3 ways to improve your study habits

How well you learn is often directly related to how hard you try. All the natural intelligence in the world won't help you if your study habits are making it hard for you to concentrate. That's why it's so important to set yourself up to succeed. As a famous motivator once said: "People don't plan to fail. They fail to plan."

Following these steps will make it easy for you to set up, and stick with, any learning schedule.

Plan carefully before starting. Setting up a good work environment before beginning is essential. Find a special area in your home where you can work. This will help you stay focused on your studying.

When you sit down to work, don't stress out about how much you have to do. Instead, try to have fun with it. Make sure you're comfortable. Study for short stretches and take frequent breaks. Rewarding yourself with a snack after 30 minutes of concentration is a good way to motivate yourself.

Stay on course. Now that you've gotten off on the right foot, stick with it. The best way to keep yourself on course is to keep your goals in mind. Do this by making lists of what you want to accomplish and then sticking to them. Don't make these lists in your head. Write them down and mark off each item as it's finished. It's amazing how encouraging it is to cross off the items that stand between you and success. Keeping these "to-do" lists also combats the tendency to waste time at the beginning of a study session wondering where to start.

While you are studying, think about how you are benefiting from this learning. Remembering why this learning is important to you and what you stand to gain from success can help keep you motivated.

Determine the next step. Like any ongoing project, the point of learning is continuity, or "stick-to-it-iveness." Always be thinking about what the next step of your learning journey will be and how you will take that step.

One way to keep moving forward is to offer yourself little rewards for doing well. Give yourself some time off or permission to do something fun that gets you away from your work.

It's also important to leave your workstation neat. Coming back to a mess is a discouraging way to start your next session. If you are forced to reorganize and clean up before getting down to business, you'll waste valuable time.

Besides, taking a few moments to straighten up at the end of a session allows you to go over what you've learned, reinforcing the information you need to keep. Also think about how well your studying went and reflect upon ways to do better the next time. Taking a few minutes to evaluate yourself and what you've learned can make all the difference in deciding what comes next in your learning process.

New challenges sharpen your thinking

Scientists studying the human brain have made many remarkable discoveries — thanks to the help of an order of Catholic nuns in Minnesota called the Sisters of Mankato. Their contribution to the study of the brain is very important. Since many of the sisters live well into their 90s, they are an excellent source of information on how learning affects the brain into the later years.

Researchers have been "picking their brains" for years, and the findings are amazing. Because of their healthy diet, their low levels of smoking and drinking, and their constant attention to education and learning, the sisters suffer very low rates of Alzheimer's and other types of dementia, stroke, and other brain disorders often associated with aging.

The studies also show that the nuns who are more intellectually active — those who teach, study, or do challenging mental tasks — live longer than the nuns who perform mostly physical labor.

To keep your mind sharp, here are some things you can do:

Challenge your brain. Your thought processes depend on the neurons in your brain and the connections between these neurons. The more you use your head, the more these connections have a chance to grow, expand, and strengthen. Just about every major brain malfunction, from Alzheimer's and stroke to trauma and senility, is caused partly by the breakdown of the neuroconnectors in the brain.

Like the Sisters of Mankato, you should strive to challenge your mind in every way you can. Learning something new keeps your mind active, which causes those brain building blocks to grow and "keep you connected." Mental exercises, like brain twisters and riddles, are great ways to exercise your brain.

Focus on variety. Keep your mind active in many different ways. When you force your mind to work in ways it's not accustomed to, researchers say, the activity causes growth in new and different parts of your brain. That's a good reason to try as many mental sports as you can. Here are some great suggestions.

- **Take a class.** The subject doesn't matter. Just choose something you're interested in but don't know anything about.

- **Learn a new skill.** It doesn't matter what skill you learn as long as it's new. The best skills for improving your mind, experts say, are those that require you to use your brain, your hands or feet, and your skills of coordination, like learning a new dance or exercise routine.

- **Be curious.** Make it a point to be outgoing and interested, always ready to try something new. Curiosity is the force that drives us to discover new facts, skills, talents, and people.

- **Read.** This is good for keeping yourself informed and entertained, and it stimulates your mind. Reading something completely unfamiliar to you makes it more challenging. And being well read helps you interact with others who are seeking good conversation.

- **Solve riddles.** Riddles, puzzles, mind games, crosswords, and brain teasers are great ways to encourage your brain to see things from a new perspective. (See if you can unravel the mystery of the jugs in Brain boosters at the end of this chapter.)

Welcome learning's side effects. Keeping your mind in tip-top shape has some pretty interesting side effects you should be aware of. Constant learning will make you a sharper, clearer thinker. You'll be more on your toes, open-minded, and eager to explore new things. You will be more interesting and more interested in the world around you, and you'll have more fun.

Like a physical exercise program, keeping your brain well conditioned is a process that builds on itself. The more faithfully you stick to it, the less you will want to live without it.

Keys to improving your concentration

"I want to get this done, but I just can't seem to concentrate." Sound familiar? Everyone has trouble focusing from time to time. Maybe the subject isn't something you're crazy about. Maybe you have a lot of other things on your mind. Or maybe you're just tired and would rather go to bed. Lots of obstacles can come between the things you need to learn and your ability to focus on them. But they don't have to if you remember these two important keys to keener concentration.

Key #1 — Attention without tension. Too often, you sit down to take care of business with a lot of extra baggage in your head. In order to concentrate, you need to get rid of everything else first. The best way to do this is to approach your task when you are well rested and not worried about other things.

You can also keep the tension out of your study time by keeping up with your studies. But if you have been procrastinating, don't try to catch up all at once. Giving yourself realistic goals makes the task less scary. Hunger, fatigue, and physical discomfort can also cause tension.

Key #2 — Short and sweet. How long can you concentrate? Eight hours in a row? Six? Surely, at least two? Sorry. The truth is, most people can effectively concentrate for about 35 minutes. After that, your ability to stick with the subject begins to fall off as your mind wanders and you get sleepy or bored.

Knowing your limits is a good starting point for any venture. If you are studying for pleasure, 35 minutes a day is a good, but not intimidating, commitment. If you have a lot of work to do, breaking it down into 35-minute sessions makes it easier to schedule the rest of your day.

Finally, and perhaps most importantly, when you concentrate in 35-minute bursts, instead of long, drawn-out marathons, your mind is forced to continually revise and review what it's soaking up. Most people wait for the end before reflecting on what they've learned, summing it up and storing it. When you have frequent ends, every 35 minutes, you are constantly reviewing and reflecting on your subject. You are able to summarize your learning in much greater detail and with much better results.

> *"Kindness is more important than wisdom,*
> *and the recognition of this is the beginning of wisdom."*
> — Theodore Isaac Rubin

Simple tips for super studying

What can I do to make myself learn faster? Are there skills I can work on that will help me learn more, spend less time at it, and remember it better?

Those are tricky questions to answer because everyone learns at their own pace and in their own way. For instance, you might like to read books about the brain while relaxing in your favorite easy chair, a little classical music playing in the background. Yet, your spouse might prefer sitting up straight at a desk. If he needs total silence to concentrate, that soothing classical music could very well drive him nuts.

You are unique. You'll have the most success if you don't try to conform to any set formula but rather do things that feel comfortable and natural for you.

Nevertheless, there are some tips that seem to help a majority of people. Why not try a few of them and see what works for you?

Preparation. To get the most out of your studying, take the time beforehand to get ready.

- Review what you already know about the subject. Think about how you can use this knowledge to help you learn more. Reinforce what you already know.

- Outline what you expect to gain from the subject. Think about what you expect to learn, and try to predict how it will turn out.

- Prepare to succeed by committing to success. Remove obstacles that could disturb you while you are trying to learn.

Concentration. Whenever you are actively learning, whether practicing a skill, reading, or listening to a lecture, it's important to focus on the task at hand.

- Be excited about your subject.

- Immerse yourself in the subject while you are studying.

- Keep guessing at what you'll learn next. Make predictions and see if they turn out. If you choose right, the validation will excite you. If not, evaluate what made you predict incorrectly.

Absorption. Many of us forget most of what we learn, for various reasons. Either we have too much on our minds, the subject matter was dull, or we weren't really paying close attention in the first place. Yet, there are ways around this short-term memory bogeyman. The key is to take just a few minutes of time after the fact to commit what you've learned to memory.

- Think of ways you could profit by what you've learned and write them down. You are more likely to remember things that are, or can be, useful to you.

- Think of the most positive thing you just learned — anything funny, interesting, surprising, or memorable. Why is this interesting, funny, or memorable to you?

- Think of the most negative thing you just learned. Anything that seemed stupid, doubtful, or made you angry. Why didn't you agree with this?

By finding ways to spend time with the subject matter after the fact, you naturally commit the high points to memory. This strategy of preparing, concentrating, and reflecting on the material makes you focus on the subject for an extended period of time. This strong focus leads to thought and improvement, and it's the kind of dedication that will boost your learning power.

How to make learning fun

It's no great secret that the things you do best are probably the things you love. With the possible exception of employment, no one ever put much time into mastering a subject or a skill he didn't like. In fact, people who enjoy their jobs tend to do them much better than people who don't.

Study what you enjoy. Pursue the subjects that entice you, make you laugh, raise your passions. Unless required by an outside force, like school or a job, there's no reason to spend your time learning about things that don't interest you. And if you are, for some reason, required to bone up on a subject that is boring you to death, you should probably reconsider why you are doing it. There's probably a better line of study or employment for you.

For a jump-start on a new learning experience, try this exercise. Go to your favorite bookstore or library and browse until something strikes your fancy. Don't settle for the books lying around your house. The chances are you've either read them before, or they aren't very interesting to you. If they were, you would have read them by now.

When you're trying to decide what book to grab, pick a subject you really want to know more about. The point is to make learning fun. Paying attention to what fascinates you takes the pressure off learning. After reading your new book, read it again. Or go back and get another book on the same subject, one with a slightly different approach or viewpoint.

Why do people get bored and stop reading, studying, and exercising? Because they get trapped in the same old rut. They forget to be curious. With today's multi-media and expanding educational horizons, there's no excuse for this happening to you.

A good way to keep on learning is to be curious. Let your imagination wander and wonder, and if you see something interesting, follow up on it. When you hear an unfamiliar name of a faraway city, check the atlas to see where it is. When you see a brief TV report on an interesting subject, go get a book at the library to learn more. Look up new words in the dictionary.

By staying curious throughout your life, you'll never miss an opportunity to learn something new, hear a good joke, or see something magical.

Learn the art of asking questions

As soon as you were old enough to put words together, you probably asked things like, "Why is the sky blue?" "Is Santa Claus real?" Or the ever popular, "Where do babies come from?"

Questions are the most direct path between ignorance and information, a fact that every child learns quickly. So why do so many adults shy away from this valuable tool? The answer is embarrassment. Many people are embarrassed to admit to others that they don't know something. As a wise man once said, "The only stupid question is the one that's never asked."

Don't be afraid to ask questions. In fact, whenever you're at a lecture, in the company of an expert, or in a situation where questions are welcomed, make it a point to ask at least one question. Putting yourself in the questioning frame of mind will keep your thoughts focused on the parts of the material you don't understand. If you can't think of even one question, you probably have a pretty solid grasp of the subject.

Good questions can boost your learning process. Just follow a couple of simple rules.

Ask the right questions. When you have an opportunity to ask questions, don't waste time by asking about information that could be acquired in another way. Use this chance to draw out facts or insights that would not be available in books or other resources.

If you are at a lecture or presentation, make sure you pay attention. Don't let thinking about your own questions get in the way of hearing what is being said. Asking a question that has already been answered is a waste of time.

Ask the right person. Don't ask an English teacher for tax advice. Don't ask a mechanical engineer what that pain in your ear might be. These might seem like silly examples, but it's important to know who you are talking with before asking questions. Someone who produces movies about outer space might know absolutely nothing about astronomy.

Double-check answers. Don't assume just because someone is a history professor that he knows everything about history. Unfortunately, some people like to pretend they do and would rather give an answer they're not sure of than admit that there's something they don't know. Going back and re-checking answers is a good way to reinforce correct information and reject information that is wrong.

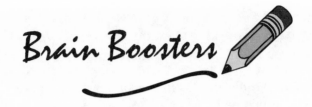

Measuring with 3 jugs

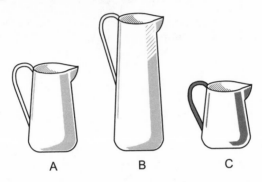

A   B   C

Using jugs A, B, and C with the capacities shown in the table, how would you measure out the volume of water indicated in the right-hand column?

With the first problem, you have a 21-cup jug, a 127-cup jug, and a 3-cup jug to measure out 100 cups. You may fill or pour out as much water as you'd like, using any of the jugs.

Find the solution to all seven problems.

Problem	Given jugs of these sizes			Measure out this much water
	A	B	C	
1	21	127	3	100
2	14	46	5	22
3	18	43	10	5
4	7	42	6	23
5	20	57	4	29
6	23	49	3	20
7	15	39	3	18

Syllabaloo

Find a word that fits the clues. The number of blanks equals the number of letters, and the numeral in parenthesis tells how many syllables make up the word. As an additional help, all the syllables for all the words can be found, given in alphabetical order, at the bottom of the puzzle.

1. One thousand years (4) _ _ _ _ _ _ _ _ _

2. Huge (3) _ _ _ _ _ _ _

3. Red bird (3) _ _ _ _ _ _ _ _

4. To come behind (2) _ _ _ _ _ _

5. Tropical fruit (3) _ _ _ _ _ _ _ _ _

6. The act of noticing (4) _ _ _ _ _ _ _ _ _ _ _

7. Strange, odd (3) _ _ _ _ _ _ _ _

8. Tools and other gear (3) _ _ _ _ _ _ _ _ _

9. Heart doctor (5) _ _ _ _ _ _ _ _ _ _ _ _

10. Act of gratitude (3) _ _ _ _ _ _ _ _ _ _ _ _

Syllables:

ap car car cu di di e fol gan gi giv gist ing len liar low
ment mil nal ni o ob ol pe pine ple ser quip thanks tic
tion um va

Check your answers in the *Solutions to Brain boosters and teasers* section at the back of the book.

Personality

How it affects your health and happiness

A popular song from the '50s goes something like this: "...'cause she's got personality, walks with personality, talks with personality ..." Terms like "personality plus" and "lots of personality" are usually compliments. They make the assumption that personality means a "good" personality. Saying someone has no personality usually means the speaker finds the other person boring and uninteresting. But everybody has personality of some kind — whether it's bold or shy, softhearted or tough, serious or silly.

Your personality is what sets you apart from other people. Your mood may change from day to day, even moment to moment. But personality is the way you think, feel, and act day in and day out, over a long period of time. It includes your feelings, attitudes, and ways of looking at the world.

A wide variety of personality types have been described by different kinds of psychologists. You're probably familiar with the type A and type B personalities and how they relate to health. The type A personality represents the hard-driving workaholic that drops dead of a heart attack at age 45. The type B personality represents the laid-back happy-go-lucky person who never worries about anything and lives to be 101.

There are some problems with such a simplistic view of personality and health. The vast combinations of personality traits are too complex to be broken down into two simple stereotypes. However, stereotypes often contain a kernel of truth. Research finds that your personality and how you deal with stress can indeed affect your health, but few people fit the type A or type B profile all the time. Most fall somewhere in between.

Personality tests like the *Meyers-Briggs Type Indicator* offer a more in-depth look at personality types. These are often used in career counseling and in business. Employers use them to understand the preferred working and communication styles of employees.

Workers take a test and are then labeled as a type, like "feeling" or "thinking," an "S" or a "C," a "golden retriever" or a "beaver," a "blue" or a "gold." All descriptions are presented in mostly positive terms. One type isn't considered better than another. But some are more suited than others for different types of jobs. These tests also give employers and coworkers more information on how best to interact with each other.

But some people think these tests are given more credibility than they deserve. A report from the National Research Council finds the popularity of these tests "troublesome" because they haven't been proven to work.

No matter what any tests say about your personality, you are a unique individual. Learning to understand your personality traits and how they relate to your health may benefit you mentally, emotionally, and physically.

How to take control of your life

Would you describe your personality as a hardy one? If so, you are probably a pretty healthy individual as well. Psychologist Suzanne Ouelletes Kobasa studied business executives who stayed healthy despite the stress of running a company. She identified three traits of these people who have a "hardy" personality:

Commitment. The healthy executives felt a commitment to themselves and to what they were doing. They knew what their priorities were and were comfortable talking about what was meaningful in their lives. They exhibited curiosity about life and wanted to give their energy to living it fully.

Control. A feeling of control contributes to the hardy personality. They have a sense of being able to make decisions that make a difference, while others may just passively follow orders. Other studies find that nursing home patients who are allowed some degree of control, such as being allowed to arrange their personal possessions and choose their daily activities, become more alert, happier, and healthier.

Challenge. Hardy people take on life with enthusiasm and energy. They thrive on change and are eager to face new situations.

The executives in Dr. Kobasa's study who didn't fall into her "hardy personality" category were more likely to experience illness regardless of their age, income, or job level.

If you don't think your personality fits into the three Cs, commit yourself to the challenge of taking control of your life. You might just cut your doctor bills in the process.

The way you dress: It's all in your 'genes'

Stand on any street corner in any city, watch the people go by, and you'll see some really strange clothing. Do you ever wonder why some people dress so weird? According to research, it may be their genes.

Researchers have identified a gene that contributes to "novelty-seeking," that personality trait that drives people to try new and different experiences, sometimes to the point of endangering their lives. This gene is probably shared by skydivers, bungee jumpers, and yes, weird dressers.

A recent study found that people who scored high on tests of fashion innovation also scored high on tests of sensation seeking. People who wear unusual, flamboyant clothing may just be engaging in a less risky form of novelty seeking.

The next time you spot someone on the street with purple spiked hair and orange eye shadow, try to be understanding. It's much safer than skydiving.

Banish illness with a positive personality

"Calm down, you're going to have a heart attack."

"Don't worry so much, you'll give yourself ulcers."

These common statements show that many people believe your personality can affect your health. The idea of a connection between personality and health isn't a new one. More than 2,000 years ago, Hippocrates believed that certain personalities were more likely to develop heart disease. Today's research shows evidence that the father of modern medicine was correct about heart disease. Links with personality and cancer, asthma, ulcers, and other disorders have also been suggested. There even seems to be a general disease-prone personality.

Heart disease. Probably the most well-established link between personality traits and a physical disorder involves your heart. Several studies have found that traits of the "type A" personality, particularly hostility and anger, are associated with a higher risk of heart disease. A recent study found that another personality trait, submissiveness, may also be linked to heart disease, but this time favorably. People who were considered submissive according to a psychological test were less likely to suffer non-fatal heart attacks.

Ulcers. For years, people have believed that worry was the cause of ulcers. People who were under emotional stress would begin to suffer stomach pains, and sure enough, soon they'd be diagnosed with ulcers. However, in 1982, research uncovered a tiny, spiral-shaped bacterium named *Helicobacter pylori* (*H. pylori)* that is now accepted as the main cause of ulcers. Still, the belief that personality contributes to ulcers persists. Perhaps it's because many people report feeling worse when under emotional stress. So although your personality may not cause you to develop ulcers, it may contribute to them.

Asthma. People with asthma seem to share certain personality traits, including anxiety and a powerless, out-of-control attitude. But it's uncertain whether these personality traits contribute to asthma, or whether suffering from asthma brings out these traits in people. It is most likely a cycle, with the disease causing anxiety, which in turn makes the asthma worse. Regardless of which causes the other, controlling your anxiety may help lessen asthma symptoms.

General illness. Some researchers say there is a disease-prone personality. Certain combinations of personality traits may cause someone to be more susceptible to all kinds of disorders. One study found perhaps the most revealing trait shared by people with a "disease-prone" personality. They reported feeling more emotionally stable when they were ill.

Don't accept the fact that your personality will cause you to develop a disease. There is no evidence that any personality trait can directly cause you to become ill. However, combined with other risk factors, your personality may make you more vulnerable. Follow the suggestions in the following story and the *Emotions* chapter for the best ways to make your personality a healthy one.

"You can't have any effect on the cards that you are dealt,
but you can determine how you play your cards."

— Milton Erickson

Secrets to a stress-free personality

You have a great personality. Everybody says so. Your personality makes you who you are, and you wouldn't want to change that. However, research finds that your personality can have a profound effect on your health.

The main culprit in the personality/health connection is stress, which releases hormones (cortisol and adrenaline) that are designed to help you deal with adversity. However, too much of these hormones can be damaging.

Everyone has stress in their lives, but the key seems to be in how you deal with it, and that's where your personality comes in. You may deal with pressure differently than someone who is more or less outgoing, expressive, or emotional.

Knowing what stresses your type of personality may help. A test designed by True Colors, a personality consulting firm, identifies not only what type of personality you are, but also what stresses your type. If you know what kind of situations place you under too much pressure, you can try to avoid those situations or work to deal with them more effectively. See if you can recognize your personality and identify your stressors.

Gold personalities like things neat and organized. They are practical and dependable; prepared for every situation. They like to have clear-cut procedures and routines to follow every day. What stresses gold personalities:

- disorganization

- constant change

Blue personalities aren't necessarily sad people, despite their title. They are very loving, caring individuals who avoid conflicts. They always consider the feelings of other people. What stresses blue personalities:

- rivalry and competition

Green personalities think about situations logically. They are problem-solvers and are often demanding, especially of themselves. They dislike routine, and constantly strive to make things better. What stresses green personalities:

- repetitive tasks

- people who don't take their work seriously

Orange personalities are easily bored and enjoy a wide variety of activities. They are spontaneous, prone to do things on the spur of the moment. They dislike waiting and tend to be disorganized. What stresses orange personalities:

- a job with a rigid structure and organization

- any activity that keeps them from moving around.

"Such is the nature of men, that howsoever they may acknowledge many others to be more witty, or more eloquent, or more learned, yet they will hardly believe there be man so wise as themselves."

— Thomas Hobbes

When guilt is good for you

Can having a guilty personality be good for you? According to one study, yes and no. The type of guilt you feel can mean the difference between a positive or negative effect on your mental health.

The study found that chronic, ongoing guilt unrelated to specific events was associated with symptoms of depression and other mental problems. This happens to people who feel guilty even when they've done nothing wrong.

However, predispositional guilt, which is a tendency to experience guilt over specific types of events, can actually be healthy for you. In the study, those who experienced predispositional guilt were more likely to participate in volunteer work and religious activities, both of which are beneficial to your health. They were also less likely to experience hostility, which has been associated with an increased risk of heart attack.

The key to dealing with guilt may be to decide if you've actually done anything to feel guilty about. If you have, feel guilty, and then get over it. If you constantly feel guilty for no reason, you may need to see a therapist to resolve your guilty feelings before they damage your health.

Your unforgettable personality

You may be able to change your personality, but you're not likely to forget it. Studies find that people with amnesia are able to describe their personalities accurately.

One woman who suffered a concussion in a fall became unable to remember anything that had happened in her life for several years previous. However, her insight into her personality remained accurate despite her massive memory loss.

In another case, a man with permanent memory loss was still able to describe his personality similar to the way his friends described it.

Researchers think this shows that you don't have to remember how you behaved in the past to know how you are likely to behave in the future. In fact, they theorize that personality may be stored in a different type of brain system than your memory and knowledge.

So maybe you don't have to remember that you've always color-coded your clothes hangers to know that you like to be organized.

Dependability — the key to a long life

Are you a careful, conscientious person? Can your friends always count on you to do the right thing? If so, according to one study, you may reap the benefits of your dependability by living a longer life.

A long-term study that followed people for more than 70 years found that those who were rated high in dependability as children were more likely to live into their 70s. Another surprising finding of the study was that people who were less optimistic and cheerful also tended to live longer. The protective effects of pessimism and conscientiousness were about equal to having low cholesterol and low blood pressure.

This study contradicts other research that says optimism is the key to a long life. Researchers think it may mean that conscientious people are more likely to take care of themselves — having regular checkups and eating healthy — while overly optimistic people may be more likely to engage in risky activities that could cut their lives short.

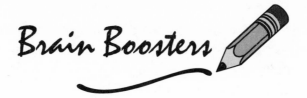

Your 'write' personality

Numerous personality tests have been designed to tell you whether you are an introvert or extrovert, intuitive or judgmental, thinking or feeling. Some people believe that even your handwriting tells a tale about your personality. People study for years to become graphologists — experts in the art of handwriting analysis.

Want to know if your handwriting reveals the "true you?" Write the following sentence on a blank sheet of paper:

I have a great personality.

Now check the *Solutions to Brain boosters and teasers* section at the back of the book for a simple description of your "write" personality.

If you enjoyed that, perhaps you'd like to try your hand as an amateur graphologist with the writing samples on the following page.

1. **Who would you hire to drive and accompany you to parties and other social events? (You want this person to fit in more as a companion than an employee.)**

Paula: *I will be a good choice!*

Angie: *I will be a good choice.*

2. **Who do you trust to pay $189 for your antique vase?**

Morris: *I will pay you $189 for the vas*

Harry: *I will pay you $189 for the vase.*

3. **Are both writers sincere?**

Becky: *I really do LOVE you*

Charlie: *Please believe I really love you.*

4. **Which person does the writer not care for?**

I spent the afternoon with Sally, Toni, and Agnes.

Check your answers in the *Solutions to Brain boosters and teasers* section at the back of the book.

Attitude

Change your outlook, change your life

"Your attitude can make or break you," the speaker advises young adults just beginning their careers.

"What it takes is a winning attitude," the coach tells his team.

"You need an attitude adjustment," says the father to the rebellious teenager.

From parents to professors, everyone has something to say to young people about attitude and success. But maybe you are not a student or an athlete. Perhaps you've passed the time of fast-track career building. So does attitude still matter?

You bet it does. Every day of your life. Your happiness, health, and accomplishments are affected by what you think and feel from moment to moment. Unfortunately, some people with a terrific attitude about the struggles of their earlier years find it harder to keep a positive outlook when facing challenges later in life.

But attitude is a choice. You can't always control your circumstances, but you can control the way you respond to them. And people who face each stage of life with a positive mental attitude are the ones who handle the stresses best.

"The greatest discovery of my generation is that human beings,
by changing the inner attitudes of their minds,
can change the outer aspects of their lives."

— William James

10 tips for a positive future

The wind was against them now, and Piglet's ears streamed behind him like banners as he fought his way along, and it seemed hours before he got them into the shelter of the Hundred Acre Wood and they stood up straight again, to listen, a little nervously, to the roaring of the gale among the tree-tops.

"Supposing a tree fell down, Pooh, when we were underneath it?"

"Supposing it didn't," said Pooh after careful thought.

An optimist like Pooh looks on the bright side of things. He gets out of bed in the morning expecting things to go well. And generally they do. That's because people with a positive outlook are likely to do things that lead to success.

If you are an optimist and you have a problem, you probably first look for a cause outside yourself. If you can't find one, you'll think of the reasons you contributed to the problem and feel confident that you can work it out and not repeat it.

On the other hand, if you are a pessimist, you generally assume that whatever can go wrong will. And you probably find lots of proof. By focusing on the negatives, pessimists seem to attract problems their way.

Optimistic people are usually persistent. They often keep going when others would quit. They combine enthusiasm with positive thinking.

But negative thinkers blame themselves for problems. Instead of looking for a solution, they dwell on their feelings of worry, shame, hurt, or anger. If there's any chance things won't work out well, they are likely to give up in frustration. "Why bother? Nothing ever turns out right for me."

A touch of pessimism isn't necessarily a bad thing. The blind optimist may cheerfully ignore signs that a problem is brewing. By the time he takes action, it may be too late. But you can balance your positive attitude with a healthy dose of realism without dwelling on the negatives. Taking the day-to-day problems of life too personally isn't healthy. Most research shows that if you are an optimist you'll have fewer illnesses and may live longer than those who are pessimists.

Although you may have learned most of your attitudes in childhood, don't despair. You can change your thinking at any age. Here are 10 easy ways to develop a more positive view of life.

Practice smiling. It helps you feel more upbeat and encourages you to see things in a positive light.

Expect the best in every situation. You won't find the evidence of the bright side if you aren't looking for it. Believe you can reach your goals, then take steps each day to make them happen.

Be open to new ideas. Don't rush to make judgments before hearing all the facts. Try stepping outside a situation to get a different point of view.

Involve yourself with positive, capable people. And don't let yourself feel threatened by their accomplishments. Rather see your association with winners as a sign of your own worth.

Be friendly. Let others see that you respect and appreciate them. They, in turn, are more likely to show you the same respect.

Trust yourself to master challenges. Assume no one is coming to rescue you, but you can do it for yourself. Don't look for someone to blame when things don't work out. Instead take responsibility and make needed changes.

View your mistakes as opportunities to learn. Did you know that if you started a business that failed, you'd find it easier to get a start-up loan for a new venture than you did the first time? If you have faced defeat yet have the enthusiasm to try again, you have certainly learned from your mistakes. So bankers view you as a better credit risk.

Bounce back quickly from bad circumstances. Acknowledge your pain and frustration. Then put your focus on a plan of action and move forward to better times.

Share the credit when things go well. A generous attitude of appreciation increases the likelihood of continued success.

Look for inspiration from positive thinkers. Consider this true story. During the 1960s, a merchant became quite successful importing a bright new cloth from India and selling it to clothing manufacturers. But soon they began returning all the items made with the cloth because it faded so badly. He tried unsuccessfully to make it colorfast, but nothing worked. He was about to go bankrupt when he decided to change his approach. He advertised the material as guaranteed to fade. From this came the fad of wearing clothes of faded madras plaid.

Cure illness with this powerful health booster

What you believe is true can have a powerful effect on what you experience. Consider this example, reported in the *British Medical Journal:*

A construction worker jumped down on a large nail. He was in great pain when he arrived at a hospital emergency room. Even the smallest movement hurt so much medics had to give him a sedative before they could examine his foot. On removing the boot, they saw that the nail had gone between his toes. There was no injury.

This is a clear example of the power of belief. Fortunately, the opposite can happen too, like when a mother kisses a "boo-boo" and the child, believing it will heal, forgets the hurt and runs off to play.

How else does your mind affect your health? Some experts say that 60 to 90 percent of the time you go to a doctor it's for something that can't be helped by medicine or surgery. If you trust your doctor's reassurance that it isn't serious, you'll probably feel better right away.

But you may think only medicine will make you better. So your doctor, knowing that what you think affects your health, may prescribe a placebo. Although this is a pill that has no active medicine in it, you are likely to get better anyhow.

Then there are other times when you expect something to get worse or to hurt, like the man with the nail in his boot, and it does. This is called the nocebo effect. The word placebo means pleasure. Nocebo is the opposite.

Many people think the placebo effect works only with conditions that are "all in your head." But research shows they can be effective with conditions like high blood pressure, heart problems, asthma, and ulcers.

Herbert Benson is a medical doctor who has written books about the connection between the mind and body. He believes that when you expect your body to be healthy it responds with better health. Instead of "placebo effect," he likes to call it "remembered wellness."

If you are like most people, you are healthy most of the time. Yet you may fear some dreadful illness or disease is just waiting to get you. That's understandable with so much emphasis on illness all around you, especially in the media. Advertisers in particular encourage your concerns about your health. They know that fear sells products.

It's easy to forget the amazing ability your body has to heal itself. So when you feel bad, you may think you need some kind of treatment. The placebo pill or your doctor's reassurance that all is well triggers the body to respond to "remembered wellness."

Benson suggests that, even when your illness requires medical treatment, you try to focus on the things that are going right. To the extent that your health and other problems will allow, pay attention to the people and situations that make your life good.

This takes the focus off the pain and illness, giving your body the best chance to remember its natural strength and vitality. Your "remembered wellness" helps you get better.

Say 'no' to negative thinking

If your next-door neighbor passes you in the shopping mall and doesn't speak, how do you feel? Well, it probably depends on what you think.

If you assume she didn't see you, you may feel disappointment. If you think she's distracted by a problem, you'll probably feel sympathy. If you think she is deliberately snubbing you, you might feel anger. If you remember that you forgot to return a book you borrowed, you may feel embarrassed and relieved that she didn't see you.

Your beliefs don't change the reason for your neighbor's not speaking. But they do determine your feelings and maybe your actions as well. If you automatically assume the worst, you may invest a lot in negative emotion for no good reason. And you may do things to make matters worse.

If you continually have negative thoughts, you may suffer from depression. If that is the case, you might enlist the help of a cognitive therapist. Cognition means "thinking." This kind of therapist is trained to help you spot negative thinking and to help you see things more realistically.

Maybe you aren't depressed but sometimes let negative thinking create problems. If you'd like to be more positive in a given situation, change your thinking and you'll change your experience.

- Begin by paying more attention to your thoughts. Notice when your beliefs and attitudes are negative.

- Ask yourself why you think things are the way they are. Do your negative beliefs stand up under the light of reason? If not, what would be a better attitude?

- Regularly ask yourself if there is a better way of seeing things. Think of someone you admire. What would that person think and do in a situation that you find bothersome? What would be your best advice to a friend who had the same problem?

You may find it hard to get in the habit of examining your thoughts this way. But chances are, the pleasant emotions that follow will be well worth the effort.

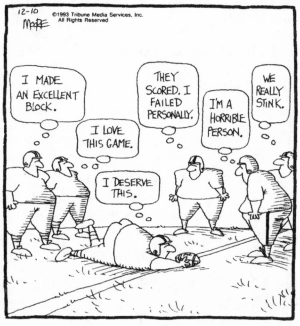

Reprinted with permission.

A dozen ways to boost your self-esteem

When you meet new people, do you feel confident they'll like you? Do you look forward to learning a new skill, expecting to pick it up quickly? Do you know what your strengths are? And do you feel comfortable with your weaknesses? If you answered yes to these questions, you probably have high self-esteem.

When you have a positive self-concept, you see yourself as a good person. You usually feel well balanced and generally comfortable with your physical, mental, social, emotional, and spiritual health. You likely find your strengths buffer you against life's difficulties.

If, on the other hand, you lack confidence in yourself, you probably avoid situations where you might expose your weaknesses. This may mean you hold back in any situation where there is a chance of failure. And that includes a lot of life since risks are a natural part of almost any success.

There are many advantages to having high self-esteem. When you feel good about yourself:

- the world seems a happier place.

- you are less likely to use drugs.

- you take better care of your health.

- you'll have fewer ulcers and sleepless nights.

- you're more apt to persist at difficult tasks.

On the other hand, if you have low self-esteem, you experience the opposite. And you are likely to feel more unhappiness and despair when things go wrong than other people do in the same situation.

Most people with low self-esteem have an internal critic that constantly puts them down. ("What a dummy I am. No wonder no one likes me. I always mess up. I can't seem to ever do anything right. Way to go, stupid.")

Self-talk can be a self-fulfilling prophecy. You convince yourself it's true, so you continue to do things that reinforce that belief. Here are 12 positive ways to avoid self put-downs.

Practice interrupting negative self-talk. Pay attention to what you say about yourself. When you catch yourself being critical, respond by saying something like, "Stop this nonsense right now!"

Write down your self-criticisms. Invest about 15 minutes a day for a couple of weeks. Write out all the negative things you catch yourself saying. Then write what is true. For example:

- Critical voice: "I never do anything right."

- Response: "That's ridiculous. I make some mistakes, but I do lots of things right."

Remind yourself of what you lose. A negative self-concept can make it hard to try new things that you might enjoy because you think you'll fail. You may lack the support of friends because you hesitate to take the risk of rejection. Making a list of all the things you miss out on can motivate you to pay attention to your self-talk.

Surround yourself with positive encouragement. Put up little signs where you'll see them. "Jack, your kindness to others shows what a good person you are."

Look for people who feel good about themselves. They'll be good models of high self-esteem. Avoid those who think putting others down is "cool."

Practice positive self-talk. Stand in front of a mirror. Look yourself in the eyes and say, "I'm really a good person, trying to do the best I can. And I'm getting better every day. As a human being, I am allowed to make mistakes. I feel just fine about that."

Write letters of appreciation to yourself. Commend yourself on any job well done. (Dear Joy, I liked the way you talked to Anne about her rose vine invading the yard where the grandkids play barefoot. You asked her nicely to come clip them. You thanked her when she agreed and accepted her apology for not realizing they were a problem. Way to go, Joy!)

Visualize your success. Imagine other people complimenting you on things you do well. These can be real accomplishments or things you are working to achieve.

List your strengths and celebrate them. Remind yourself daily of your good qualities. (I am a warm and caring person. I have a really good sense of humor. I keep my promises.) Maybe even make up a song about yourself and sing it every day. Give yourself a treat to honor your specialness.

Be honest about your weaknesses. Decide where you could use some improvement. Be accurate but not judgmental. Decide what you can do, then do it.

Practice integrity. Identify your highest values and try to live by them. The closer you follow your ideals, the better you'll feel about yourself. But practice patience. The strongest and wisest sometimes fall short.

Look for the best in others. When you get in the habit of noticing the good qualities of others, perhaps you will be reminded of your own good traits as well. For one week, try to treat everybody you meet as someone special. See how they act. When you show others your sincere respect and appreciation, they are more likely to do the same to you.

"It's surprising how many persons go through life without ever recognizing that their feelings toward other people are largely determined by their feelings toward themselves, and if you're not comfortable within yourself, you can't be comfortable with others."

— Sydney J. Harris

The life and death P.O.W.er of initials

William Owen Wilson and Virginia Irene Potts are probably proud to carry monogrammed luggage. And they probably like to wear their initials, W.O.W and V.I.P., on their clothing as well. On the other hand, people with initials that spell P.I.G. or Y.U.K. are less likely to advertise these acronyms that invite jokes and put-downs.

The initials you carry throughout your life may do more than determine whether you get admired or ridiculed. They may affect how long you live. Dr. Nicholas Christenfeld, a researcher at the University of California at San Diego, has found a connection between positive and negative initials and longevity.

It seems that Mr. Wilson, with the acronym W.O.W. to keep him inspired, would likely live four-and-a-half years longer than someone whose initials spell a neutral word or one that has no meaning. But Patrick Isaac Green, with the initials P.I.G., would be likely to live almost three fewer years. Christenfeld found that suicides and accidental deaths — both believed to be associated with psychological problems — were higher for those with negative initials.

So if you're naming a child, you may want to think about the long-term effect of his initials. An A.C.E. or J.O.Y. might do very well in life, but a B.U.M. or R.A.T. may already have the cards stacked against him.

The secret to a peaceful mind

Where do attitudes come from? Perhaps your negative thinking can be traced to your childhood. Other attitudes you picked up somewhere along the way. Thinking about past problems can be good if it helps you change unhealthy behaviors. Beyond that, it's best to just let it go.

Focus on what you can do in the present to handle today's concerns. A "that was then, this is now" attitude is most helpful to finding peace in your life.

During times of stress, even happy times, it's not uncommon for self-confidence to suffer and a negative attitude to creep in. This was true for a Georgia woman named Jane. The night before her daughter's wedding, Jane spent a sleepless night. She was happy for her daughter, but her mind was filled with angry thoughts toward her ex-husband.

At the rehearsal party, he had breezed in to play the devoted father-of-the-bride. The groom's family had obviously found him charming. But Jane kept remembering all the times he had been absent when their daughter had really needed him while growing up.

Although she tried to put angry thoughts out of her mind, she just couldn't seem to let it go. She worried that she would not be at her best for her daughter the next day, but angry thoughts continued to intrude and keep her awake.

In her desire to ensure a happy day for her daughter, Jane questioned why she was so angry at this late date. She had to admit that with her daughter now leaving home, she had some doubts about the kind of mother she had been. By dwelling on the faults of her ex-husband, she had made him into the bad parent. And, by comparison, she saw herself as the good parent.

On realizing this, Jane got out of bed and found a sheet of paper. Following the advice of experts, she made two columns. In the first, she listed all the ways she had done well by her daughter. On the other, she listed her shortcomings. When she compared the two, she realized she had by far done more right than wrong. And on examining the list, she saw a couple of negatives that still could be changed. She determined that she would, at the appropriate time, set those things right.

No longer angry, she went to sleep. The next day, having finally rested well, Jane thoroughly enjoyed herself and was cordial to her ex-husband. The wedding photographs gave no hint of the turmoil she had felt the night before.

You can't change the past. But you can control how you think about it. And remember, attitude is contagious. When you choose to be happy, it helps those around you to be up-beat as well.

> *"The day the child realizes that all adults are imperfect,*
> *he becomes an adolescent; the day he forgives them,*
> *he becomes an adult; the day he forgives himself, he becomes wise."*
>
> — Alden Nowlan

How to get the most out of your goals

If you have set goals and reached them, you probably view your life as successful. But studies show that just having and pursuing goals can make you feel healthier and emotionally satisfied whether you reach them or not. That is, if they are the right kinds of goals.

Life-task goals. These are the general, long-term goals you are committed to accomplishing. Life-task goals that promote feelings of closeness to others will bring you the most satisfaction and well-being. On the other hand, working toward a goal of controlling, manipulating, or impressing others may bring you negative feelings and emotional distress.

Achievement goals. There are two kinds of these specific short-term goals — mastery goals and performance goals.

- **Mastery goals** are those in which you strive to get better at something or to master new skills. People with mastery goals usually work hard to reach them. They are generally self-motivated. When they face challenges, they work harder to achieve success, and their performance usually improves as a result.

- **Performance goals** are those that call for a positive response from others. People who strive just for approval often suffer anxiety and tend to have lower self-esteem. They are more likely to fear failure and so not attempt more difficult tasks. Even though their intelligence may be equal or superior to others, they may be perceived as less capable because they find it more difficult to gain new skills and show them.

Intrinsic and extrinsic goals. The passion to do something just because you want to comes from intrinsic desire. If you "follow your bliss," as mythologist Joseph Campbell put it, you will find more excitement and creativity in what you do. And since you are more likely to stay enthusiastic, you have a greater chance of succeeding.

To do something for profit or recognition, or to avoid punishment, is an extrinsic goal. Like the performance goals, these depend on rewards coming from others. People who focus on extrinsic goals are more likely to lose interest and find less pleasure in their pursuits.

Your health and well-being are affected by your behaviors. It's never too late to choose new goals. When you choose the healthier ones, your behaviors will change for the better as well. Your rewards will include better mental and physical health.

*"Everything can be taken from a man but one thing:
the last of the human freedoms — to choose one's attitude in any given
set of circumstances, to choose one's own way."*

— Victor Frankl

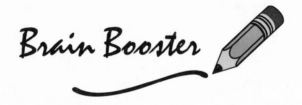

Attitude cryptograms

Can you break the code of these cryptograms? Each is a quote having something to do with attitude. To figure them out, you must determine which letters of the alphabet have been substituted for the correct spellings. Each quote has a different code.

Example:
BVAOVAX IDE OVPJZ IDE RFJ DX IDE RFJ'O —— IDE FXA XPTVO. — VAJXI WDXH

Solution: Whether you think you can or you can't — you are right. — Henry Ford

1. SULJOSW OE WUUB UQ MCB MKL LJOSHOSW ICHTE OL EU. — ZOPPOCI EJCHTEDTCQT

2. PWHJ VMT ABB HKS WBHO SBGBKSA H XMMS SBHQ MK PWBOB VMT HOB AJHKSYKX; YJ HQAM SBGBKSA MK PWHJ AMOJ MN GBOAMK VMT HOB. — D.A. QBPYA

3. ZSP LHPRZPH ARHZ JK JMH SRAADEPVV JH XDVPHN CPAPECV JE JMH CDVAJVDZDJEV REC EJZ JMH IDHIMXVZREIPV. — XRHZSR FRVSDELZJE

4. NJM IRE IJXFORDE APIRMVP HJVPV SRQP ZSJHEV, JH NJM IRE HPTJDIP APIRMVP ZSJHEV SRQP HJVPV. — GDLLN

5. ORJ JHJ LJJL ZUEH NRBO ORJ XWUC WL GPJGBPJC OZ MZXGPJRJUC. — RJUPW IJPVLZU

6. YL-LOHPXCL HBB MWJ AHSL ELLC VWBQ ... QXIPXII FAHV XCIJBVI MWJY IWJB. — FHBV FAXVPHC

Check your answers in the *Solutions to Brain boosters and teasers* section at the back of the book.

Mindpower

Using your brain's full potential

Your amazing brain has the power to do even more than store "book learning" and help you make wise, well-thought-out decisions. In fact, it does some of its most important work when you don't have time to think. But sometimes using it too much can be bad for you. Your brain function can suffer, for example, if you're dealing with constant stress. You might forget things more easily and find it harder to concentrate.

On the other hand, you can use the tremendous power of your mind to improve your thinking skills. You can change habits, overcome phobias, increase your athletic abilities, and even strengthen your immune system. In this chapter, you'll learn ways to tap into these abilities to reach greater success in all areas of your life.

> *"This time, like all times, is a very good one,*
> *if we but know what to do with it."*
>
> — Ralph Waldo Emerson

Learn to ace life's stress tests

Imagine coming home alone in the dark. Opening the door, you find an intruder lurking in the shadows just a few feet away. Your heart starts pounding, your blood pressure skyrockets, and your breath comes out in short gasps. You feel yourself dripping with sweat as your muscles tense in preparation to either fight or run away.

In times of danger, your brain quickly barks out orders to the rest of your body to prepare you for action. This is what we call the "stress response." And these changes occur whether the threat is real or imaginary. If the stranger in the shadows turned out to be a raincoat and hat hanging on a coat rack, you'd still feel these same physical sensations.

Stress can shrink your brain. If you are in real danger, the stress response can save your life. But if you call on it too often and for long periods of time, it can kill your nerve cells. Amazingly, research with monkeys shows that the brain may actually create new cells to replace them. Unfortunately, it doesn't seem to restore lost cells as long as the stress is still going on.

Prolonged stress is bad for you, plain and simple. It keeps your brain from learning and storing memories. It weakens your resistance to illness and may lead to emotional problems. And it can make it harder for your body to repair itself after an injury.

So it's important to recognize situations in which the stress response will help. But it's also necessary to know when it's best to remain calm.

Confidence can help lower stress. Your ancient ancestors ran into their caves to avoid wild beasts. Later on, a duel with pistols was a quick way to settle disagreements. But today's stresses are often more complex. You are apt to bring on more trouble when you try to run away from family problems, for example. And it certainly doesn't help to get into a fistfight with your boss or with someone who cuts you off in traffic.

Fortunately, your ability to use your brain has increased. Now you have more options for handling stress than simply running or fighting. By thinking ahead and making quick adjustments, you can avoid a lot of difficulties. You can talk your way out of others. The more confident you are that you can handle a problem, the lower the stress will be.

But in this busy, modern world, you can't avoid stress altogether. And who would want to? Life could get pretty dull if everything always went smoothly. But not all stresses are exciting challenges. Some are unwanted and difficult, yet unavoidable. It's good to know you can learn techniques that make them a whole lot easier to handle.

How to stay in control. In the 1970s, a lot of doctors were concerned about the effects of stress on the heart. So Dr. Herbert Benson and his associates at Harvard University decided to study the claims of people who were practicing meditation. They found that, indeed, their blood pressure, heartbeat, and respiration did slow down. In fact, they discovered everything that increased with stress, decreased during meditation.

Since what they found was the exact opposite of the stress response, Benson called these changes "the relaxation response." Based on this research, he developed a simple meditation almost anyone could do. He wrote a book about it called *The Relaxation Response*. Meditation, however, is only one of several ways you can reach this state of relaxation.

Many universities, hospitals, and health clinics are teaching relaxation techniques. These are meant to complement traditional health care, not replace it. But, as you know, lowering stress goes a long way toward preventing and treating a lot of problems.

The good news is that not only can you lower stress while you practice relaxation, but afterwards you can handle a lot more hassles before your brain and body get stressed out again.

You can learn most of these techniques without a teacher if you are patient and really practice. Devoting 20 minutes twice a day while learning is ideal. Most people find that setting a particular time and place helps them get into the relaxation habit and stick to it. The progressive relaxation technique on page 159 is good to learn first. You'll find it helpful when used alone or in combination with one of the others.

Stress test

How much stress have you had in your life recently? To get an idea, take this stress test. Circle the LCU (life change units) number following any event listed that you experienced during the last year. Then add up all the circled numbers.

A score between 250 and 500 is moderate. If your score is higher, you face the risk of stress-related problems. So be sure to read the stress management information in this chapter carefully.

Life change event: LCU

Health	Score
An injury or illness which:	
kept you in bed a week or more or sent you to the hospital	74
was less serious than above	44
Major dental work	26
Major change in eating habits	27
Major change in sleeping habits	26
Major change in your usual type and/or amount of recreation	28
Work	
Change to a new type of work	51
Change in your work hours or conditions	35

Changes in your responsibilities at work:

more responsibilities	29
fewer responsibilities	21
promotion	31
demotion	42
transfer	32

Troubles at work:

with your boss	29
with co-workers	35
with persons under your supervision	35
other work troubles	28

Major business adjustment	60
Retirement	52

Loss of job:

laid off from work	68
fired from work	79

Correspondence course to help you in your work	18

Home and family

Major change in living conditions	42

Change in residence:

move within same town or city	25
move to a different town, city, or state	47

Change in family get-togethers	25
Major change in health or behavior of family member	55
Marriage	50
Pregnancy	67
Miscarriage or abortion	65

Gain of a new family member:

birth of a child	66

adoption of a child	65
a relative moving in with you	59
Spouse beginning or ending work	46

Child leaving home:

to attend college	41
due to marriage	41
for other reasons	45
Change in arguments with spouse	50
In-law problems	38

Change in the marital status of your parents:

divorce	59
remarriage	50

Separation from spouse:

due to work	53
due to marital problems	76
Divorce	96
Birth of grandchild	43
Death of spouse	119

Death of other family member:

child	123
brother or sister	102
parent	100

Personal and social

Change in personal habits	26
Beginning or ending school or college	38
Change of school or college	35
Change in political beliefs	24
Change in religious beliefs	29
Change in social activities	27

Vacation	24
New, close personal relationship	37
Engagement to marry	45
Girlfriend or boyfriend problems	39
Sexual difficulties	44

Personal and social

"Falling out" of a close personal relationship	47
An accident	48
Minor violation of the law	20
Being held in jail	75
Death of a close friend	70
Major decision regarding your immediate future	51
Major personal achievement	36

Financial

Major change in finances:	
increased income	38
decreased income	60
investment and/or credit difficulties	56
Loss or damage of personal property	43
Moderate purchase	20
Major purchase	37
Foreclosure on a mortgage or loan	58

Total score: _____

Reprinted from the *Journal of Psychosomatic Research, Volume 43, No. 3*, Miller and Rahe, "*Events and 1995 LCU values for the RLCQ*," pages 291-292, 1997, with permission from Elsevier Science.

Easy does it with relaxation training

What scares you most, seeing a snake or taking a test? In either case, just relax. Your test scores will improve, and those serpents won't seem so scary. A study of college students found that those who practiced relaxation had significantly higher test scores than others in the study.

And for phobias, it's not just a snake-oil treatment. In a study of people who had an extreme fear of snakes, those who learned relaxation techniques were able to voluntarily get closer to caged snakes than those who didn't have the training. Their heart rates were slower, and they felt less fear than the non-relaxed participants.

You can put panic in its place with relaxation training. In a study at Stockholm University in Sweden, half of those who were prone to panic attacks practiced relaxation while the other half learned how to change their thinking about the attacks, a practice called cognitive therapy.

Both groups made tremendous improvements right away. And a year later, not only were there no relapses, but 55 percent of those who had panic attacks right after training no longer experienced them.

Other research shows that relaxation can have a positive effect on the immune system of cancer patients, even while undergoing chemotherapy. And people with depression may improve more with relaxation than with medication. This is also true for folks with high blood pressure.

Progressive relaxation is a powerful, yet simple, process. You can practice it lying down or sitting up. Here's how:

- Choose a quiet, comfortable spot.

- Take a few extra-deep, slow breaths.

- Close your eyes and progressively relax your body one muscle group at a time. Start by clenching the muscles of your toes to tighten them while you count to 10. Then relax them for a count of 10. Do the same with the muscles of your feet.

- Continue up your body, tensing and relaxing each muscle group. By the time you reach the top of your head, all the tension in your body should just melt away.

"Nothing in all creation is so like God as stillness."
— Meister Eckhart, 13th century

Meditate for mindpower

You may think meditation is some kind of unusual, far-out religious practice. But over the last 20 years or so, research shows all kinds of people have been enjoying its benefits.

In one study researchers were able to predict higher scores on intelligence tests by how long the person had been meditating. And a study of older meditators (average age 81 years) found improvements in learning, speaking, and thinking. Their mental health was better, and they felt more in control of their lives. After three years, their survival rate was about 94 percent, much higher than for the non-meditators in the study.

You might find meditating keeps you out of the doctor's office. If you look at insurance statistics comparing meditators to non-meditators, you'll see quite a difference. The two groups get about the same amount of health care for childbirth. But in 17 other categories the meditators require 30 to 87 percent less medical attention. Think of the time and money saved. Meditating for 20 minutes may look more attractive with those numbers!

Researchers believe meditation can be especially helpful in preventing and treating heart disease. A 1996 study found that meditators did better on exercise tolerance tests. Other research shows it reduces blood pressure and cholesterol, both high risk-factors for heart disease.

Meditation also helps relieve chronic pain, anxiety, and substance abuse. And it has helped Vietnam veterans with post-traumatic stress syndrome. If you're interested in discovering the benefits for yourself, here are a couple of methods you can try.

Relaxation Response. When Dr. Benson developed this meditation, he wanted it to be acceptable to all people, regardless of their religious beliefs. So he suggested you choose a word or expression that has a special meaning to you. You might use a word that reflects the feeling you want, like "peace" or "joy." Or you might repeat a prayer or verse of scripture.

To practice the relaxation response:

- Get in a comfortable position.

- Close your eyes, breathe deeply, and relax your muscles as you learned with progressive relaxation.

- Now concentrate on your word, phrase, or prayer. Let all thought fade away. When other thoughts intrude, gently come back to this focus.

- Continue to repeat this word or words for 10 to 20 minutes.

Mindfulness meditation. Do you spend so much time worrying about the past or being anxious about the future that you can't deal with what you're facing today? If so, maybe mindfulness meditation can help you put things in a better perspective. Mindfulness is about focusing on what's going on right now. After all, the only time you can change anything is in the present.

People who practice mindfulness believe that paying attention to your breath helps you become more in touch with other experiences of your life as they are happening.

To practice this form of meditation:

- Relax and follow your breath in and out. Pay attention to the beginning, middle, and end of each in-breath.

- Do the same with each out-breath. Notice the rise and fall of your chest or abdomen. Don't try to breathe any differently from your normal breathing.

- Continue breathing slowly and evenly for 10 to 20 minutes.

'Raisin' your awareness

Do you sometimes treat yourself to your favorite candy bar, only to realize half-way through that you hardly noticed eating it? If you were eating "mindfully," this wouldn't happen.

Students in a stress-reduction class at the Community Health Center in Meriden, Conn., learn "mindful eating" as an exercise in focusing on the present. The instruction goes something like this:

- Hold a single raisin in the palm of your hand, and observe it carefully for a few minutes.

- Imagine you are seeing a raisin for the first time. Notice its appearance – the color, shape, wrinkles – and the way it rests in your hand.

- Think about how it grew on the vine as a grape; how the sun, rain, and soil nourished it. Imagine how it was picked and dried in the sun.

- Place the raisin in your mouth. Feel its roughness against your tongue.

- Bite into the raisin, focusing on its sweet taste. As you chew, notice the changes in the texture.

- Pay attention to the sensation of slowly swallowing it. Does the flavor linger in your mouth afterwards?

Mindful eating is probably much better for your digestive system. And it may lead to more focused attention on other everyday activities. Perhaps taking a bath or washing the dishes could become a richer experience if you do it mindfully.

Imagine a richer life

Are you a daydreamer? Do you like to replay a story you've read or a movie you've watched over and over again in your mind? Perhaps you've lingered over the romantic words a sweetheart wrote and felt the same swell of emotion that accompanied the first reading of those lines.

Is daydreaming a waste of time? Maybe not. Salesmen use their imagination to their advantage every time they mentally rehearse a sales presentation. Athletes do the same when they visualize a perfect pitch or swing. Each time a student recalls the look of admiration on the teacher's face when handing back a test with a big "A+," she is increasing her chances that it will happen again.

Unfortunately, people often spend much of their time imagining the worst without realizing they are setting themselves up for failure. By mentally rehearsing positive outcomes, you can change a negative habit and enjoy greater success. The key is to turn daydreams into action by planning and guiding them to meet your goals.

Most people find imagery works best if they combine it with relaxation. They use this combination to increase confidence, self-esteem, and emotional well-being, and reduce anxiety and depression.

In a study where people practiced imagery before abdominal surgery, they reported less pain afterwards. They felt better able to cope with the pain they did have, and they required less medication.

People with cancer can successfully use imagery and relaxation to regain lost weight and to relieve pain, stress, and the nausea of chemotherapy. In one study of people hospitalized with cancer, 92 percent reported positive results with relaxation therapy. Studies also show improvements in their immune system.

Research even shows nursing mothers can double their milk production with mental imagery. And people with glaucoma use it to reduce the symptoms.

Mental imagery (or visualization) isn't limited to just *seeing* with your imagination. Some people are not as visual as others. But you can use any of your senses — hearing, touching, even smelling or tasting. Maybe when you use your imagination, you just have a *feeling* of something happening. However it comes to you, your imagination can do some important work.

The process of visualization is simple:

- Get in a comfortable position, either sitting or reclining.

- Follow the process of gradual relaxation.

- Imagine scenes that you find relaxing. This alone produces health benefits because it reduces stress.

- Be more specific by imagining what you want to create in your life. Observe yourself giving a speech with confidence, for example. Or maybe you want to practice making perfect moves on the basketball court.

You can watch yourself leaving a health clinic after chemotherapy, smiling and relaxed. Continue imagining yourself going through your day, comfortable, energetic, and happily spending time with family or enjoying a hobby.

Whatever your need, use your imagination to help create it. When you think of things you fear, visualize their opposite. If you worry about traffic accidents, for example, imagine yourself cruising calmly and safely through heavy traffic. The more you do this, the more it will become a habit. You'll find yourself practicing it in your daily life without necessarily having to set aside a special time.

Can meditation lower the crime rate?

Has your temper ever gotten you into big trouble? Meditation is a good way to reduce anger that gets out of hand. People at the Center for Mindfulness in Medicine, Health Care, and Society at the University of Massachusetts Medical Center teach prison inmates mindfulness meditation. They find it lowers hostility and raises self-esteem.

A California study followed 259 male parolees who had learned and practiced meditation while in prison. When they got out, they committed fewer repeat crimes than those who did not meditate. Five years after parole, their rap sheets showed meditation did more to reduce returns to prison than education, vocational training, or psychotherapy.

You may find your anger gets you into more trouble with relationships than with the law. But meditation can keep you cool where you once might have gotten hot under the collar. And who knows? It just might keep you out of jail.

No-fail technique for self-improvement

You may know you have a really sharp brain. But procrastination, a lack of self-confidence, or maybe a fear of test-taking keeps you from advancing in your career. Maybe you are too shy or nervous to speak up about what you want in a relationship. Or you may lack the energy to handle all your many responsibilities. Never fear. Hypnosis can come to the rescue.

Psychotherapist Kenneth Scroggs, director of the Northpines Center in Norcross, Georgia, has been helping people improve their lives with hypnosis for more than 20 years. His advice is to take what you already know and let hypnosis help you improve on it.

For example, oversleeping is making you late for work. You *know* what you need to do, but you just can't seem to do it. Instead of getting up when you hear the alarm clock, you turn it off and go back to sleep.

But you can use hypnosis to fall asleep faster and to sleep better. It can help you get up feeling rested, wide awake, and enthusiastic about your day.

"On a deeper level," says Scroggs, "your subconscious mind really wants what is best for you. It's concerned about your basic survival and your happiness. Hypnosis allows you to form a direct partnership with your brain. It helps you cut through distractions and anxieties to make better choices."

When some people think of hypnosis, they imagine dimly lit rooms, smoke and mirrors, con artists who take your money, or worse. They think a hypnotist can trick you into doing things against your will. But the truth is, that image of hypnosis belongs in the movies, or maybe on the stage where an entertainer uses showmanship and cooperative people from the audience for a fun demonstration.

Research shows that hypnosis is a respected tool for self improvement. And whether directed by a therapist or practiced as self-hypnosis, you are always in control. All hypnosis, when you get right down to it, is self-hypnosis.

Hypnosis begins with relaxation and imagery and adds a third element — suggestion. When you are relaxed and focused, your critical mind is less active. So positive statements you make while under hypnosis have a powerful effect. These statements are called post-hypnotic suggestions.

Scroggs stresses the importance of planning to get the results you want from each session. "Be very clear about what you want to visualize and what your suggestions will be once you are under."

He often suggests to clients that they write out their script and record it, playing some pleasant, relaxing music in the background. He says, "If they are really committed to success, they usually don't mind the extra trouble."

If you write it out, you can go over it and be sure your suggestions are clear and positive. Then you can record it, reading slowly. Just start the tape, relax, and let the sound of your own voice take you deeper than you might go if you were having to remember what to say.

Here's the three-part process of self-hypnosis that Scroggs teaches. After you've read through it, you can decide if you want to tape it or not.

Relax your body and mind. "I find that if people go too slowly, they fall asleep or get distracted. So I have developed a way to help my clients get into the hypnotic state more quickly," says Scroggs.

He divides the body into three parts: toes to waist, torso plus arms and hands, and neck and head. He teaches his students to select a word to associate with a different kind of relaxation for each area.

To relax the lower part of the body (toes to waist), choose a word that suggests a comfortable physical sensation like "warm," "cool," "light," or perhaps "heavy," unless you are working on weight loss. "You could choose "numb" if you are using hypnosis for dentalwork or childbirth," suggests Scroggs.

Let's say you choose "warm" as your key word for physical relaxation. Start with three deep, slow breaths. Then let your attention move to your toes. Say, "My toes are now relaxed and warm." Imagine the feeling of warmth in your toes.

Continue with, "My feet are now relaxed and warm." As you relax your calves, thighs, abdomen, hips, and buttocks, associate the word and feeling of warmth. When you reach you waist, take a deep, slow breath and say, "I am now completely relaxed and warm."

According to Scroggs, after some practice, you can quickly relax the lower part of your body by saying the word "warm" and imagining the feeling of warmth. "The brain learns through association and repetition," says Scroggs.

The second area of the body, between the waist and neck, is more related to the emotions. (Think of a mother cuddling a nursing baby or love represented by the heart.) For this area choose a key word like "peace," "joy" "love," or "calm."

Again, take three deep breaths as you prepare to relax emotionally. As you relax your diaphragm, chest, back, shoulders, arms, and hands, repeat a statement as you did with the first part. ("My chest is relaxed and I feel calm.") When all of these muscle groups are relaxed, say, "I am now completely relaxed and calm."

Take three more deep, slow breaths as you get ready for the last stage of relaxation, the mental relaxation. Scroggs says, "Slowing your breath slows your brainwaves and your heart rate. This slows down your thinking and helps you focus better without distractions."

As you relax the muscles of your neck and head, begin to associate relaxation with a special place rather than a word. It could be any place you think of as a place to relax. You might choose a secluded beach or your favorite easy chair.

Imagining yourself in the special place, begin to relax your neck. Pay special attention to releasing stress in the muscles on the sides as well as the back of your neck. "Relaxing these muscles," says Scroggs, "prevents headaches that tension in this area often causes."

As you relax your jaw, let it drop slightly so there is a little space between your top and bottom teeth. As you relax your face, forehead, temples, and scalp, continue to imagine yourself in your special place. Say to yourself, "I am now warm, calm, and completely relaxed."

"Some people like to do a little check at this point to show they are really under," Scroggs says. "Say to yourself, 'I am so relaxed that my eyelids want to stay closed. Even if I tug on them gently, they just want to stay closed.' Reach up and check this out. Don't force your eyes open. Let it be a gentle checking."

As you move into the next phase, visualizing your special place, say gently to yourself, "Let go, let go, let go."

Imagine a special place. Scroggs suggests you try to involve as many of your senses as possible. If you are at the beach, imagine the warmth of the sun, the sparkle of light on the waves, the cool breeze, the sound of seagulls, even the taste of salt on your lips. In your easy chair, imagine the warmth and firmness of the support beneath you. You might imagine the scent of roses from your garden drifting through an open window, or soft music playing on your radio.

When you have spent a while creating and enjoying your special place, say positive things to yourself like, "My life is happy, and I enjoy good health." Or, "My energy and enthusiasm for life get stronger every day."

Imagine yourself going through your normal daily activities with the same happiness and enthusiasm. Then imagine yourself in the situation that you want to change or improve. But now imagine the positive scene that you planned in advance. Remember to use as many of your senses as possible for the best results.

Give yourself positive suggestions. Now you are ready to add your suggestions to the imagery. Scroggs says to be specific and realistic. He suggests, "Rather than 'I want to be a millionaire,' or even, 'I will make lots of money today,' try, 'Today I will really enjoy eating the lunch I take to work to save money.'"

Always use clear, positive statements and images of what you want. Avoid negative suggestions. Words like "no" and "not" don't bring up images or feelings, so you might miss them in the hypnotic state.

For example, if you want to lose weight, say, "I am completely satisfied eating a healthy salad for lunch today." Imagine yourself biting into crisp greens and juicy tomatoes. See yourself chewing slowly, enjoying the flavors and textures. Imagine the feeling of a comfortable fullness in your stomach as you push away from the table with a smile of contentment.

If you say, "I will not eat chocolate cake today," you may have suggested and given a clear picture of yourself eating chocolate cake. So remember, keep the suggestions positive. State what you want to be true. If a picture of a tempting piece of chocolate cake enters your mind, visualize pushing it away and reaching again for that delicious salad.

An interesting thing about visualization under hypnosis is that an impossible fantasy scene works just as well as a realistic one. A man with back pain visualized the computer-game character Pac-Man moving back and forth across his back, eating up excessive pain. And it worked!

One warning: Be careful about how you use self-hypnosis for pain. You don't want to substitute pain control for treatment of a serious condition. Think in terms of easing or managing pain, rather than getting rid of it completely, unless it's for something temporary like dentalwork or childbirth.

When you have completed your imagery and your suggestions, prepare to return to your normal awareness by taking three deep, slow breaths. Say positive things to yourself like, "Every day I feel better and better about myself. My self-hypnosis is getting faster and deeper. I now return to my normal awareness feeling relaxed and energetic. My mind is sharp, and I am now wide awake, wide awake."

Let yourself ease back to normal alertness. Allow yourself time to slowly become aware of your usual surroundings. Take your time in getting up and moving about.

Be patient with yourself if you don't get dramatic results right away. Just continue to practice, remembering to keep your attitude positive. Eventually your success may amaze you.

Try biofeedback for proven mindpower

Do you like the idea that you can influence your body with your mind, but you actually need to see it to believe it? Well, some people will tell you you'll see it *when* you believe it. After all, positive thinking is an important step in improving your life with mindpower.

But if it helps, you can have the proof right before your eyes. You can use a biofeedback device to show that your blood pressure really does come down, for example, when you use imagery or hypnosis for that purpose.

In the 1960s the term "biofeedback" was first used when people were trained to change their heart rates, blood pressure, and brain activity. Before then people didn't believe you could voluntarily control those functions.

Any gadget that gives you information about your body — a thermometer or your bathroom scale, for example — could be called a biofeedback device. More advanced biofeedback machines include the EEG (electroencephalograph) to monitor brain waves and the EMG (electromyograph) to measure muscle tension.

Biofeedback is used to treat, among other things, migraine headaches, digestive disorders, high blood pressure, chronic pain, heart rhythm abnormalities, Raynaud's disease, and epilepsy.

Biofeedback can also help speed the healing of wounds. In people suffering with foot and leg ulcers, the healing rate was 10 times faster for those using biofeedback to increase blood flow to their feet and legs.

Are chronic pain and insomnia keeping you awake at night? Biofeedback can help there, too. But you may not like the idea of being hooked up to a biofeedback device. No problem. Most people find they can get just as much help from relaxation, mental imagery, or hypnosis without wires, beeping sounds, or flashing lights.

If you prefer to get proof with biofeedback, you'll need to find a trained professional to teach you what to do and to hook you up to the appropriate monitor. You'll know it was worth the effort when you get more control of your body's functions. And once you've mastered the techniques, you probably won't have to depend on the machines.

4 quick stress-busters do their job

Is your job your biggest source of stress? If you are a nurse, doctor, or other healthcare worker, chances are your answer is yes. As a result, you are more likely to suffer from anxiety, depression, chronic illnesses, and drug and alcohol abuse.

To find the best ways to combat these problems, 100 hospital workers took part in a study. They were divided into four groups that regularly spent 10 minutes doing something to bring down their stress level.

- One group received a 10-minute massage.

- A second group sat in comfortable chairs in a dimly lit room and listened to soothing music.

- Another group practiced gradual muscle relaxation and visualized pleasant scenes.

- And members of a social support group relaxed and talked to each other in an encouraging way.

At the end of the study, all four groups showed less anxiety and depression than before. They were more rested, energetic, and clear-thinking. All groups appeared to be equal in their improvements. Although researchers already knew these practices were helpful, they were quite surprised that sessions lasting only 10 minutes could be so effective.

So keep that in mind during your next work break. Maybe one of these techniques will help you return less stressed and more productive.

Designer music to improve your mind

You might think singing along with the radio is fun entertainment. And dancing to your favorite tunes may be a great way to exercise. But did you know music is good exercise for your mind as well?

If you want to sharpen your mental clarity, music can make it happen. It can increase your energy and your feelings of caring about others. It might even save your life! That's because music reduces stress, hostility, and sadness. These tend to increase your risk of heart disease and immune system disorders.

OK, so music is powerful. But, you may wonder, does all music affect you the same? No, say researchers at the Institute of HeartMath in Boulder Creek, California. That's where composer Doc Lew Childre creates "designer music" for specific effects.

The music on his album *Speed of Balance*, for example, was designed to create mental and emotional balance, to help the listener think more clearly and see things in a more positive light. And the music of his Heart Zones affects the physical health of listeners.

In a recent study, Childre's *Speed of Balance* was compared to selections of grunge rock by Pearl Jam, New Age songs by Enya, and classical pieces by Mozart. The designer music had, by far, the most favorable influence on listeners.

Researchers looked for the positive effects of mental clarity, relaxation, vigor, and caring. They also checked for negative emotions: hostility, tension, fatigue, and sadness. Designer music increased all the positives and decreased all the negatives. The grunge rock showed exactly the opposite — increases in all negative categories and decreases in the positive ones.

The classical music lowered fatigue, sadness and tension but made no difference in the positive effects. Listening to New Age music resulted in a decline in caring, mental clarity, and vigor, as well as in hostility and tension. The only increase was in relaxation.

So pull on your best designer jeans and dance to some designer tunes. It'll do your mind and body good.

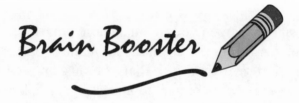

Awareness check

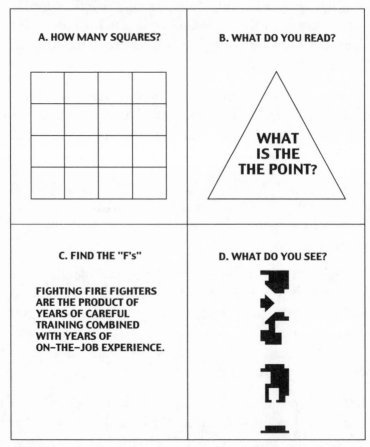

Sometimes our minds see things that aren't really there or miss things that are. Give your mind an "awareness check," and see if it's on the ball.

Wakeup Calls: You Don't Have to Sleep Walk Through Your Life, Eric Allenbaugh, Discovery Publications, 1992

Check your answers in the *Solutions to Brain boosters and teasers* section at the back of the book.

Emotions

The 'heart' of the brain

Sing and dance with joyful laughter. Weep with the grief of a broken heart. What would life be like without emotions, those feelings of the heart?

Some people think it's far superior to act from logical thinking rather than from your feelings. And it's true. Acting too quickly based on your emotions might get you in trouble — like when you respond with a quick temper to something someone says.

But a person with high-intellectual intelligence can make poor decisions in his personal life. A wise balance of IQ (intelligence quotient) and EQ (emotional quotient) is more likely to lead to happiness, health, and success in life.

Give your feelings a face lift

When you are feeling down, it can help, as the song says, to "put on a happy face." Research shows that going through the motions can stir up the emotions. If you smile, especially if it's a full smile where you raise your cheeks, you really will feel happier.

By the same token, if you force a frown, you'll feel worse. And if you furrow your brow, you'll feel sadder. The feelings will follow the actions. This may surprise you. Most people think they change their expression after they feel the emotion, not the other way around.

Our facial expressions help us communicate. Look at the following drawings and see how quickly you can identify which is happy, sad, mad, and scared.

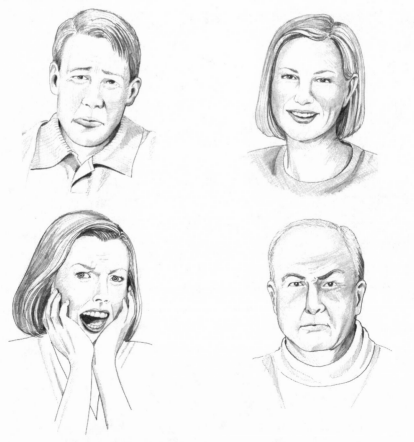

Pretty easy, right? You can probably recognize another's feelings at a glance.

Showing emotions probably helped your early ancestors survive. Nature invested a lot in the ability to make faces. Of the 44 separate facial muscles, you use only four for chewing. You use the rest for expression — 15 of them just to laugh.

And what shows on your face is evident in your body as well. When actors in a study held a fearful expression for 10 seconds, their heart rate increased by eight beats per minute. When they made an angry face, they increased both their heart rate and finger temperature. So if you are a "hot head," you really do "lose your cool."

If you want to feel what others are feeling, smile or frown along with them. But sometimes that's easier said than done. What if you walk into a room and find your best friend laughing and crying at the same time? Should you put on your best expression of sympathy, or laugh along with her?

How is it possible to be both happy and sad at the same time? It's because you process positive emotions, like love and happiness, in the left hemisphere of the brain. And you process negative ones, like worry and sadness, on the right side. This means both can go on at the same time.

Sounds are another way of changing your mood. Saying *e* and *ah* makes you smile and feel better. Maybe that's why you squeal "Wheee" when riding a roller coaster. And it could explain why it feels so good to say "Ahhh" after a big sip of your favorite, thirst-quenching beverage. But you'll feel worse if you say the German letter *ü*. That's a good reason to avoid the sound you might make when looking at something really yucky.

How you move can also affect how you feel. Notice what it's like if you shuffle your feet and look down when you're walking. Then see what a difference it makes to take long strides, swing your arms, and look straight ahead.

Pay attention to your voice and body language. Not only can it improve your communications, it just might make it more fun to go to amusement parks.

"There is a split between intelligence of the heart and of the intellect. They have to be brought back together if our children's future, and our very society are to survive."

— Joseph Pearce

Getting in touch with men's feelings

Women sometimes complain that men just don't show enough emotion. And some men prefer it that way, thinking women are too emotional. But that's not how life starts out. At birth and for the first six months or so, boys are more excitable and express more emotion than girls.

Many parents, however, are likely to train little boys out of this tendency. They discourage "unmanly" expressions, like sadness and fear. They encourage little girls, but not little boys, to express feelings of warmth and affection.

As children get older, friendships reinforce their early training. Boys more often play in larger groups with structured activities that require rules, teamwork, toughness, and competition. Girls are more likely to play with one or two other girls in activities that teach cooperation and consideration for the feelings of others.

Psychologists wonder if this may have something to do with why more men than women have problems with substance abuse, violence, suicide, accidents, and stress-related fatal diseases. And the strain on men who may feel they aren't masculine enough can cause anxiety, depression, and heart disease.

Fortunately, research about the effects of emotions on men's health is bringing more attention to this issue. For information on how to help yourself, or a man in your life, express emotions in a healthy way, be sure to read the rest of this chapter, especially the sections on anger, road rage, crying, and grief.

3 tips for a happier life

Almost everything you do is colored by how happy or unhappy you feel. Cheer up, and your relationships, your self-image, and your hopes for your future will all seem brighter. You'll feel safer, make decisions more easily, and report greater satisfaction in all areas of your life.

How happy are you? Abraham Lincoln said that most folks are about as happy as they make up their minds to be. Maybe you are one of those people who were just born happy. But some people, it seems, really do have to work at it. Could it be the ability to see the sunny side is in your genes?

Evidence seems to show that genes account for about 50 percent of your sunny outlook. But the other half comes from influences in your environment, including your own efforts. A 1997 survey found some interesting, and perhaps surprising, data about Americans and happiness:

- 80 percent of all Americans say they are happy.

- 90 percent rated their marriages as happy. And those who were not completely happy in their relationships tended to believe they could do something about it.

- 84 percent of those who were working said they liked their jobs. And among those who didn't particularly like their work, most felt confident they could get other employment.

Be thankful for what you have. Let's assume, based on the survey, you are already pretty happy. How can you improve your life even more? Winning the lottery? A promotion at work? Better health?

Maybe. At least for a little while. In truth, if you get those things, the increase in happiness may be temporary. Most people think more money would make life better. But the average American living in the 1990s was twice as rich in buying power as in the 1950s, but no happier.

And people who win the lottery express greater happiness for a while. But check on them a year later, and you'll find their contentment isn't much higher than it was before winning.

Enjoy the little things. You may wonder what would make you happy if your biggest wishes never come true. It's the day-to-day little pleasures, according to experts like Robert Ornstein, Ph.D., and David Sobel, M.D. In their book, *Healthy Pleasures,* they say when we look back on our lives we tend to remember the big events, like our wedding day or a promotion. But it's really things like playing with a child or taking a walk on a sunny day that give us a moment-to-moment sense of contentment. The more of those little joys you experience, the happier you tend to be overall.

Why spend your life waiting to win the lottery or become president of the company? Ornstein and Sobel suggest you fill your life with meaningful work and lots of little pleasures. Start by slowing down and noticing the little things you already do to make your life more satisfying. Keep doing those and add others.

Look on the bright side. Ornstein and Sobel also suggest you avoid being too much "in touch with reality." They find that the happiest people are optimists, folks who expect the best and don't dwell on evidence to the contrary. In other words, they're not worriers.

This doesn't mean you become mindless in the pursuit of happiness. Happily ignoring a health problem, for example, isn't smart and can lead to a lot of misery. And blissfully ignoring other kinds of problems doesn't bring long-term contentment either. In fact, happy people will tell you some of the greatest joys of life come from what you do to help others with their difficulties.

Mail some merriment

Are you one of those thoughtful people who cheerfully spends the time, money, and effort to send greeting cards on holidays? If so, you may sometimes wonder if they really brighten up life for those who receive them.

According to researchers at Penn State University, Christmas, Hanukkah, and New Year's cards really do make people happy. In fact, the more holiday cards people get, the stronger their feelings of well-being.

In this study, most greeting cards seemed to come from old friends — people the recipient hasn't seen for at least a year. And these messages hold special meaning for people of all ages.

For older folks, the cards represent a link with people from the past. Being remembered serves as an affirmation of their self-worth. Younger people enjoy them as a way to build and maintain social contacts over time and distance.

What happens to these cards — do they get saved and treasured? No, most cards are thrown out after the holiday is over.

Sharpen your wit with laughter

The things that make people laugh may vary from group to group. But humor of some kind is enjoyed in all human cultures. And it's hard to think of anything we do that brings more benefits.

You may think improving your thinking is no laughing matter. But, in fact, humor can sharpen your brain. It helps keep you alert, increases your creativity, and improves your memory. Laughter involves the entire cerebral cortex of the brain and gives it quite a workout. From the moment someone asks, "Have you heard the one about ...?" your brain goes into action.

When you laugh, you breathe more deeply, bringing more oxygen to your brain. This makes you more alert, releases tension that blocks learning, and increases your memory.

Laughter really is good medicine for both your mind and your body. Here are more ways it can help.

- Humor encourages you to keep a positive and hopeful attitude. And if you have uncomfortable feelings related to aggression or repressed sexuality, humor can provide a guilt-free way to release them.

- People with a good sense of humor tend to have less fear of their own mortality. That may be why they are more likely to sign the organ donor consent on their driver's license.

- Humor helps you handle stress. Laughing at someone else's joke can ease tension. But if you can find something to laugh about in life's most serious moments, that's even better. Humor you create helps you see a stressful situation as less threatening.

- By sharing humorous, real-life stories, you can enhance your social relationships. This helps improve your health.

- Laughter helps your circulation by increasing your blood pressure and heart rate. This brings more oxygen and nutrients to your tissues and removes impurities, helping to fight infection.

- Chronic breathing problems, like emphysema, improve with laughter, due to better ventilation and mucus clearing.

- Quicker recovery from illness and strengthening your immune system are two more reasons for "tickling your funny bone."

- Laughing heartily for 20 minutes equals three minutes of hard rowing. That's pretty good heart-healthy aerobic exercise.

Laugh your pain away

Did you ever laugh 'til you hurt? Or hurt until you laughed? Laughter can relieve pain. In fact, some hospitals have added things like humor rooms or "comedy carts" to provide humorous materials to patients. But humor for pain relief works best if you choose your own "medicine."

In a Florida hospital, when people recovering from surgery were allowed to choose the funny movies they watched, they used less pain medication than those who didn't watch any movies. But others who saw comedies that were selected for them, rather than seeing their personal favorites, needed the most medication of all.

Live longer and grow older more gracefully

The comedian George Burns was a prime example of the latest research — a sense of humor can help you live long and age well. He lived to be 100 years old and was doing stand-up comedy routines almost to the end.

With a healthy sense of humor, you'll be better able to see the advantages that come with maturity. And you'll be more appreciative of the joys you experience over a long lifetime.

- As children grow up and leave home, as friendships change, and as neighbors come and go, a sense of humor can ease and enhance your relationships. And older couples who can laugh at themselves are happier than those who can't.

- Humor helps you be more satisfied with your living arrangements. It can even help you adjust to unfamiliar settings, like a health care facility.

- Laughter contributes to a long life by promoting your physical and mental health.

- With a sharp sense of humor, you feel in charge of your life. If you can laugh at your problems, you can learn to overcome many of them. And since losses are a part of life, your sense of humor can help you cope better with the sorrows they bring.

"Everyday happiness means getting up in the morning,
and you can't wait to finish your breakfast.
You can't wait to do your exercises.
You can't wait to put on your clothes.
You can't wait to get out — and you can't wait to come home,
because the soup is hot."

— George Burns

How to keep humor in your life

Whether smiling through tears or laughing with carefree abandon, you can be your own best medicine. Just keep your funny bone in working order.

Seek out those who make you laugh. People who find healthy humor in everyday situations are good friends to have.

Read jokes and humorous stories. Watch funny television programs and movies. With so much material to choose from, you are sure to find plenty to suit your taste.

Look for humor in your daily life. People really are funny, and so are pets — even wild life. Have you ever watched a couple of squirrels chasing each other around and up and down a tree? Or a bird trying to pull a particularly resistant string from an old rug?

Stay in touch with your childlike "inner clown." Each day, the average kid laughs 300 times, but the average adult usually laughs only 17 times. To get in touch with your silly side, wear a funny hat or a plastic flower with a hidden water squirter. Pick up some oranges and juggle them. Try walking on stilts or bouncing on a pogo stick. Laugh at yourself when you do something ridiculous. Imagine life through a child's eyes.

Is laughter always the best medicine?

Sometimes when watching your favorite television comedy you've probably laughed until tears came to your eyes. Maybe you've laughed so hard you had to hold your sides or found it hard to catch your breath. But fainted? Most people, even those who have belly-laughed the hardest, haven't had that experience.

But one 62-year-old television viewer has — three times in fact. Once his wife had to rescue him when he fainted face-down into his dinner.

And what comedy show could have caused such a reaction? Each time he was laughing hysterically at the antics of the *Seinfeld* character George Costanza, played by actor Jason Alexander.

On each occasion, he regained consciousness within a minute. Although he watched other sitcoms, only *Seinfeld* provoked the kind of laughter that resulted in fainting.

The man had a history of high blood pressure, high cholesterol, smoking, and coronary artery bypass surgery. His doctors found partially blocked arteries coming off his aorta, the main artery to the heart.

The additional pressure in his chest when he laughed reduced the flow of blood to his brain, causing him to faint. Surgeons opened up his arteries with balloon catheterization and inserted a stent to keep them open.

As a true fan, he continued to watch the program. The good news is, at the time of a follow-up appointment with his doctor, he could watch the show without fainting.

Don't get mad, get even-tempered

It's been one of those days when just about everything that could go wrong did. You were late for work, and the boss was in a bad mood. Your secretary is on vacation, and for the second day in a row, the temp didn't show up. In your frustration, you made some careless mistakes. An important project is behind schedule, and the boss is acting like it's all your fault.

But now you're home. Your understanding spouse knows how hard you work and how unappreciated you are at the office. You can let it all out, blow off some steam, but is that a good idea?

It's probably better to just let it go. Research shows that relaxing and finding distractions will put you in a better mood. Those who talk about their frustrations tend to get more negative. Instead of rehashing the past, try taking a walk or listening to some soothing music.

Yet, it isn't just your mood that suffers when you let your fury get out of hand. Anger can interfere with clear thinking. In fact, anger and hostility can shorten your life. Men who explode with anger are twice as likely to have a "brain attack," or stroke, than those who find calmer ways of releasing their anger and frustration.

But suppressing or denying your anger isn't healthy either. You may have learned as a child to hold in "bad" emotions, like anger. But suppressing it and seething inwardly can lead to high blood pressure, which can contribute to a stroke or heart attack.

A study done at the Henry Ford Hospital in Detroit showed that men with heart disease who deny their anger are four times more likely to die from a heart attack. This isn't as likely in women because they are more apt to process their emotions.

Getting angry is a part of life you can't always dodge. But you can use these tips to help manage your anger more successfully.

Avoid situations that provoke anger. Maybe you get "hot under the collar" when you're shopping. A slow-moving checkout line or an inconsiderate sales clerk can be infuriating. Keep calm by shopping during hours when stores are not so busy. The lines will be shorter and clerks less likely to be hurried and impatient.

Recognize when anger is building. Occasional anger is normal, so don't deny it or try to cover it up. If you do, it's likely to become more explosive and harmful. If you see it coming, you are better prepared to deal with it in healthier ways. So don't wait until you are "blind with rage" to decide how you'll handle it.

Diffuse anger with calming steps. It's the intensity of the angry outburst that does the most damage. One study found that people who express anger loudly, quickly, and outwardly have more heart problems. But anger that was dealt with calmly didn't do any damage. Try some deep breathing and counting to 10, or call a friend and go for a walk. Physical activity is a great way to release frustration.

> *"Anger blows out the lamp of the mind."*
> — Robert Ingersoll

Slam the brakes on road rage

Rush hour traffic can be frustrating, even if you are one of those calm souls who rarely loses your cool. For people who easily fly off the handle, driving can become a hazardous activity.

Violence on the highway is on the rise. When these incidents occur, the explanations often seem trivial — someone was tailgating or not allowing another to pass. One driver, accused of murder, said the victim almost ran him off the road. What, he asked, was he supposed to do?

Although many of the incidents involve males between the ages of 18 and 26, males and females of all ages can drive aggressively if they let their anger get the upper hand. To avoid causing or being the victim of road rage, the AAA Foundation for Traffic Safety offers these suggestions:

Avoid offending others. If you drive with courtesy, you aren't likely to attract the unwanted attention of someone who may be easily enraged.

- **Don't cut others off.** Allow plenty of room between your car and the one in front of you. Use your turn signal to let others know before making turns or changing lanes. If someone cuts you off, assume they didn't intend to offend you. Slow down and give them room to merge.

- **Don't drive slowly in the left-hand lane.** Even if you are doing the speed limit, return to the right-hand lane after passing slower traffic. You may be "in the right," but those who want to drive faster can become angry. Just move over and let them pass.

- **Don't follow too closely.** Most drivers dislike tailgaters. To be sure there's enough space between you and the car ahead, choose a road sign or another fixed point ahead. After the vehicle in front of you passes it, at least two seconds should elapse before you pass it. Don't look at your watch. Count "one thousand one, one thousand two." If you can't see the headlights of the car behind you, it's following too closely. If possible, signal, pull over, and allow it to pass.

- **Never make offensive gestures.** If someone offends you, look straight ahead and keep both hands on the wheel. Even shaking your head in anger can set off the other driver's "hot button." Adopt an attitude of "be my guest" when another driver wants the same space as you, both when driving and parking. Keep your cool and you won't be as offended by the rudeness of others.

Don't get drawn into an angry exchange. People aren't always sensible when they are mad, but it takes two to have a fight. Stay calm by reminding yourself that you want to arrive safely at your destination.

- **Give angry drivers plenty of room.** And never pull off the road to settle things "man to man."

- **Avoid eye contact.** Look straight ahead. Eye contact makes things more personal and anger is more likely to get out of hand.

- **Get help if you think you are in danger.** If you have a cellular phone, call the police. If not, drive to a place where there are lots of people around. Use your horn to get attention. Don't get out of your car if the threatening person has followed you.

Adjust your attitude about driving. If it's your own anger that causes you problems in traffic, the best thing you can do for yourself is rethink what matters.

- **Driving isn't a race with the clock.** Allow plenty of travel time to ensure stress-free trips. Breathe deeply and relax. Listen to music or a book on tape. Arrive refreshed.

- **Give other drivers the benefit of the doubt.** Try to imagine a good reason for another's bad behavior behind the wheel. Assume there's some emergency that would explain it.

- **Learn more about anger control.** If you need more than these tips to control your temper, do some further investigation. Read books or take workshops on stress control and dealing with anger. Taking positive action will help make driving safer and more enjoyable for you.

Three cheers for tears

If you get teary-eyed over a tender scene or cry over a sad story, don't be embarrassed. And if you weep like your heart is broken when a relationship ends, that may be good. Shedding tears can help you adjust to your loss more quickly.

As most healthy people know, having a good cry can be one of the best ways to express tenderness, reduce tension, and ease pain. Those who work with people in mourning sometimes say most people not only feel better, they even look better after crying.

Research shows that children who are encouraged to cry are better adjusted than children who hold back tears. They not only have fewer behavior problems, they also think more clearly. And the ability to cry continues to benefit you as the years go by.

Shedding tears can lower blood pressure. And people who allow themselves to cry have fewer ulcers and less colitis than those who don't cry. That may be, in part at least, because emotional tears remove chemicals associated with stress. Tears caused by eye irritations don't have the same chemical make up.

Women, as a rule, cry more than men. It's not just cultural, although that's part of it. Women have more prolactin in their blood than men. This hormone is associated with both tears and milk production. From birth to puberty, there is no difference between boys and girls in crying patterns. But between 12 and 18, females develop 60 percent more prolactin and begin to cry four times more often than males.

Some men think shedding tears in public is a crying shame, but even tough guys do it. Baseball's Babe Ruth cried when he shared his cancer diagnosis with 60,000 fans. And Lou Gehrig, another baseball great, wept when he said farewell to his fans in Yankee Stadium in 1939. Actor Jimmy Stewart cried when reading a poem on television after the death of his beloved golden retriever.

What do people cry about? They shed tears of sadness (49 percent), happiness (21 percent), anger (10 percent), sympathy (7 percent), anxiety (5 percent), and fear (4 percent).

While most crying is healthy, if you are crying a lot over hurt feelings, it might be a sign you need some help. You may be dealing with a profound hurt or loss of self-esteem that is triggered by the negative things people say to you.

On the other hand, if you can't cry, you might want to try to get in touch with your deepest emotions. In either case, getting help from a therapist may be a good idea.

> *"Sorrows which find no vent in tears*
> *may soon make the other organs weep."*
>
> — Sir Henry Mandsley

Dealing with grief

Eventually, almost everybody has to deal with the loss of someone or something deeply loved. When that happens, you must face what is likely to be the most difficult emotional experience — grief.

Grief is different for each person. Some people tend to hold it in, while others show it outwardly right away. However you express it, grief is never easy.

You are likely to go through different stages of grief before coming to an acceptance of your loss. You may experience numbness, denial and isolation, anger, and depression. You may feel yearning, disbelief, confusion, humiliation, shock, despair, sadness, and guilt.

It takes longer for some people to get past the intense sorrow than it does others. But in order to recover, there are certain things you must do after you get past any initial numbness and denial.

- **Release emotion.** Research shows it's healthier to cry and talk it out. Mourning is a natural process. It may involve family and friends, as well as religious or other support groups. The important thing is to express to others how you feel.

- **Take care of your health.** Eat well and get plenty of rest. Be careful not to develop a dependence on medications or alcohol.

- **Delay major life changes.** Allow yourself plenty of time to make important decisions after a loss. Those made under the stress of grief may not be best in the long run.

- **Develop new skills and interests.** Begin gradually to make changes that open new doors to new people and new situations. This doesn't mean you forget the person you have lost. It's just a way to stop focusing on the past. And it frees you to put more of your energy into the present and future.

Most people find that, in time, they are able to enjoy life once again. You may find that the wisdom you gain from suffering enriches and deepens your life. And you will be better able to help others when they experience life's dark moments.

If you have friends or family members who are in mourning, they may need your help more than you or they know. They are at a greater risk of health problems, both physical and emotional, during this time.

According to research, the risk of death doubles in the seven months to one year after the loss of a spouse — even if the survivor is young and was previously in good health. This is truer for men than for women, but both need encouragement and support during this time.

Here are some things you can do to help yourself and others:

Make contact with a call or visit. Maybe they just need a hug. Or perhaps you can help with baby-sitting or running errands.

Encourage them to grieve. Allow time enough when you are with them so they don't feel rushed. Be available and be patient. Encourage them to talk about memories and present feelings. Grief sometimes is a long process. Don't rush them to get over it.

Be a good listener. Hear what they have to say without making judgments. Offer sympathetic comments, but don't tell them how they should feel. Avoid saying, "It was for the best," or "You'll get over it in time."

Don't be afraid to talk about it. A grieving friend may feel comforted by your memories and shared sadness about the loss.

Find comfort in laughter. Even in the saddest of times, humorous situations can occur or be remembered. It's not only permissible, it's actually good for you to laugh during times of grief. It helps create emotional distance from the sorrowful event for a little while. Researchers say people who laughed most heartily in remembering a spouse who died three to six months earlier were less prone to feel anger, fear, and guilt than those who didn't laugh much. And laughter encourages others to interact with you and give support.

Encourage the bereaved to take care of themselves. And you do the same. Often helpers neglect themselves when seeing to the needs of others.

Accept your own limitations. No matter how much you care, you cannot take away another person's grief. If, as time goes on, you sense the sorrow isn't easing or is getting more intense, you may want to suggest professional help from a grief counselor.

"The world is full of suffering. It is also full of overcoming it."
— Helen Keller

Overcoming loneliness

Katherine wheeled her chair quickly around the bed in her tiny room at the nursing home where she had lived for the last 20 years.

Expertly, she tightened the corners of the sheets as she chatted away with a visitor.

Katherine smiled, her faded blue eyes twinkling above the pink-rouged cheeks on her freshly powdered face. "The housekeeping staff has so much to do, and I'm perfectly capable of making my own bed," she said.

To see Katherine in action you would never question her good health. Unless, of course, you happened to spot her popping a nitroglycerin tablet into her mouth when the angina pains started.

Katherine had every reason to be lonely. She had no family. She had outlived her husband, her only child, and all of her known relatives and old friends. But Katherine was a favorite of the staff and other residents at the nursing home. And she received regular visits from the priest and parishioners of a local Catholic church she had never attended. These friends had recently surprised her with a 91st birthday party.

Lonely? Not Katherine.

Some people can have lots of people around and still feel lonely. Others, like Katherine, thrive on whatever relationships are available — making new friends when old ones move out of their lives. And there are still others who are totally alone, yet feel no loneliness. They may, in fact, find joy in solitude.

But millions of people are lonely. Their loneliness may bring emotional pain. And it can contribute to health problems, including cancer and heart disease. Seriously lonely people don't live as long as those who are happily involved with others. Fortunately, there are things you can do to overcome your loneliness and move into a more satisfying life.

Set realistic expectations about your relationships. Maybe you are expecting too much from family and friends. Lonely people sometimes become self-absorbed and easily hurt by what others say or do. Focus instead on reasons to feel good about yourself. And change your outlook by finding ways to be more helpful to others.

Spend time alone doing things you enjoy. Many activities, like reading, are better without distractions. Think back to things you've enjoyed alone in the past and look for new hobbies as well. This will not only add pleasure to your time alone, it will give you something interesting to talk about when you are with others.

Don't push others away when things aren't going well. There's no need to give up on relationships just because there are problems. All relationships have them and can even be strengthened by working through the difficulties.

Accept the fact that some relationships come and go. It doesn't help to blame yourself or someone else when a relationship doesn't work out. Look for ways to create new relationships to fill the void. For example, set a goal of meeting at least one new person in the next week.

Don't press for intimate relationships right away. Seek out and enjoy a wide range of friendships. Be patient with yourself and take time to choose wisely.

Know that you are not alone. There are plenty of other people feeling lonely, too. Some of them are probably looking for someone like you to spend time with.

There may be times when having caring people around is not enough. What you really need is someone to talk to who understands what you are going through.

If your loneliness is related to a separation, divorce, or death, look for a support group. People who have experienced a loss like yours can do more than provide understanding. Studies show that women with cancer who participate in support groups live longer than those who don't.

And remember — pets are also good companions for people who might otherwise be lonely. They provide affection and loyalty without making a lot of demands.

Research shows that owning a pet helps lower blood pressure and reduce stress. Since these are factors in several serious health conditions, owning a pet might even help you live longer.

Variety is the spice of a longer life

Are you married? Do you interact a lot with members of your family? Do you spend time with friends, neighbors, and work associates. Are you involved with others in community projects and religious group activities?

If so, you may find it hectic running to this meeting, that job, or another church function. Sometimes it may seem to be too much. But before you yield to the temptation to cut out some of your involvements, stop and consider this — you may be adding years to your life.

Research shows that people who have many different kinds of relationships with others live longer than those whose social networks include only one to three types.

But what if you spend all your time with a large family and lots of friends. Sorry, the numbers within one group don't add up to a longer life. It's the variety that counts.

The experts aren't sure why this is true. It may have something to do with strengthening your immune system so you can resist infection. Researchers find that those with the widest network of acquaintances not only live longer, they have fewer colds as well.

'Sense'able ways to improve your mood

If you find yourself down in the dumps, maybe painting the town red would perk you up. But for the walls of your work space, try a nice blue-green. Research shows that the color of your office can affect your mood and the quality of your work. One study found that working in a red office can result in more feelings of depression, unrest, and dissatisfaction than working in a blue-green office.

But what's best for getting your work done? Those who were most sensitive to their environment performed better on office tasks in a red work space than in a blue-green one.

In a separate study, more proofreading errors occurred in white offices than in red or blue. Females in this study reported more depression, confusion, and anger in low-saturation colors, like gray, white, or beige. But males reported more of these negative moods in high saturation colors, like green, blue, purple, red, yellow, and orange.

So look around. Changing your mood and productivity may be as simple as painting your walls. And while you're at it, do a little sniffing around as well. To increase mental function and reduce tiredness, try the scent of lavender.

Wearing a fragrance can improve your emotions, too. A Duke University study found that pleasant odors improve the moods of mid-life males and females. The use of a scent reduced feelings of tension, depression, and confusion in women. Men who used colognes not only reduced those same feelings, they also reported less anger and more vigor.

This may be because the area of the brain that processes smells overlaps the area that processes emotions. When you think about it, maybe you like certain scents because you associate them with emotional memories of happy experiences.

When will this feeling end?

When you are happy, you hope it will last forever. The blues you want to lose right away. But what can you expect realistically? Here's how it usually turns out:

- Fear and disgust disappear fastest.

- Anger and guilt last a little longer.

- Joy and sadness tend to stick around the longest.

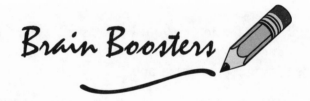

Happiness quiz

If you'd like to see how much you have in common with other happy people, take this quiz. Some of the answers might surprise you. And maybe you'll pick up some ideas about ways to bring more happiness into your life.

1. Are you male or female?

2. Are you over 50 years old?

3. Do you have close friendships or a satisfying marriage?

4. Do you usually sleep well?

5. Do you have a meaningful religious faith?

6. Do you generally feel good about yourself?

7. Is your intelligence higher than average?

8. Do you have a disability?

9. Is your income higher than that of most of your neighbors?

10. Did you have a happy childhood?

11. Have you had difficult times in your adult life that caused you great unhappiness?

12. Do you prefer taking a walk to sitting on a park bench?

13. Do you find it more enjoyable to work in your garden or go riding in a motor boat?

14. Would you rather watch a soap opera or talk with a friend?

15. Which would suit you more, reading a magazine or collecting donations for a good cause?

16. Which are you more likely to do, go to a party or stay home in case your kids call?

Rhyming pairs

Each of the following pair of words rhymes with a famous pair of people.

Example — tack and pill (answer: Jack and Jill)

1. quarrel and party

2. funny and care

3. pane and label

4. bomb and fairy

5. fan and lean

6. nick and rain

7. picky and penny

8. joy and pail

9. madam and grieve

10. duty and the feast

Check your answers in the *Solutions to Brain boosters and teasers* section at the back of the book.

Sleep

Fool-proof way to recharge your brain

Do you regularly bounce out of bed after a good night's sleep? Or does your brain feel full of fog as you drag through your day after tossing and turning all night?

At one time, people slept when it was dark and woke with the light of dawn. But the discovery of electricity means you can now work and play far into the night. As a result, a lot of people are losing sleep.

But how important is sleep anyhow? If you sleep for eight hours each night, you spend one third of your life in slumber. Is that just wasted time? Or is sleep more than just a way to rest your body?

If you think sleep isn't a matter of concern to your "gray matter," think again. Because what goes on in your brain while you slumber has a lot to do with how well you perform when you are awake.

Snooze your way to a better memory

You probably know from experience that you learn new things more easily when you are rested. But did you know that getting a good night's sleep after learning something new helps you remember it better? And if you really want to hold on to what you've learned, you need to know which nights to get the best sleep.

Learn when to sleep. The kind of memory you use to remember straight facts doesn't seem to be affected much by any particular sleep pattern. But when you learn the procedures for doing a task, the first and third nights afterward are important to remembering what you learned.

Let's say, for example, you are taking a computer class on Monday nights. You'll remember the steps in operating a new program better if you get a good night's sleep Monday night and again Wednesday night.

The second night doesn't matter so much. So if you've volunteered to stay at the hospital with a sick friend, the night to do it is Tuesday.

Slumber through stage two. For remembering new motor skills, like skating or typing, the first night's sleep is most important. You especially need uninterrupted stage-two sleep, a light sleep that occurs more in the later sleep cycles.

If you get good sleep of this kind, you'll perform the skill 20 to 30 percent better the next day than you did even right after learning it. Since stage-two sleep is strongest in the last half of the night, getting up early to practice a new motor skill, as athletes often do, can be self-defeating.

Stick to a schedule. You will also learn and remember better if you keep to a regular sleep schedule. Researchers asked students to stay awake four hours later than usual. Then they gave them tests of procedural skills (things you learn to do by practicing the steps in order). Even though they made up the time by sleeping four hours later in the morning, students didn't do as well on the tests. Experts think you remember better if you stick to the same sleep schedule after learning something new.

Remember better with REM. Throughout the night you go through a series of 90-minute cycles with different kinds of sleep in each. For remembering procedural skills, REM sleep, the kind in which you are most likely to dream, seems to be most important. REM sleep is strongest in the last hour before you wake up, so getting up early to study is not a good idea.

The secret of peak performance

Whether giving a speech, playing a game of golf, programming a computer, or teaching a co-worker a new skill, there's one secret to being your best — a good night's sleep.

When you are well-rested, you can focus your attention, hold your concentration, and remember faces and facts. You speak more clearly, are more creative, and react more quickly.

Sleep is like a tonic for the brain. But when you are deprived of sleep, your thinking ability and your motor skills get sluggish. You're also more likely to find yourself in a bad mood. Sleep loss can zap the fun right out of the things you do.

And sleeping part of the night may be worse than missing a whole night's sleep. One sleep study found that people who slept less than five hours in a 24-hour period did worse on thinking skills tests than those who had lost a whole night's sleep. They reported more negative moods as well. Researchers aren't sure why this happened but think the shorter sleep also may have been more disrupted. This happens, for example, with doctors who are on call or parents with sick children.

So if you want to be at your best during the day, make sure you get enough quality shut-eye every night.

13 ways to fall asleep faster

Good sleep is critical to the frontal area of your cerebral cortex — the part of the brain that helps you speak clearly, pay attention, and ignore distractions. This is also where you'll find your short-term memory and creative thinking. Unfortunately, it is the first area to slow down when you don't get enough sleep.

If you are like most healthy adults, you need between seven and nine hours of sleep a night. But this varies. Some people thrive on five or six hours, while others require 10 or 11 hours to be at their best.

How long you sleep often doesn't matter so much as how rested you feel. People who are satisfied with their sleep report less confusion than those who may have slept longer but more fitfully. They also tend to be less depressed, tense, angry, and fatigued.

Most sleep problems can be overcome by paying attention to your habits and making a few changes. Try these tips to help you nod off in no time.

Keep to a sleep schedule. Go to bed at the same time, even on weekends. And get up at your regular time, even if you stay up later than usual.

Don't take naps during the day. They can make it harder to sleep well at night.

Make sure your bedroom is comfortable. Most people sleep best in a room that is dark, quiet, and cool.

Leave off caffeine. Afternoons and evenings should be caffeine free. This includes coffee, tea, colas, chocolate, and some medications.

Avoid eating a big meal near bedtime. Greasy and spicy foods, especially, can keep you awake. Carbohydrates, however, may help you sleep better. A glass of milk and a bagel, or a bowl of cereal, might just do the trick.

Skip alcohol and cigarettes. A night-cap may help you fall asleep faster but can interfere with sound sleep later. Cigarettes, too, can keep you awake because nicotine is a stimulant.

Get regular exercise. But don't exercise during the three or four hours just before bedtime. Daytime exercise out of doors is especially helpful. Exposure to sunlight during the day helps you sleep better at night.

Relax quietly before bedtime. Put away your work, don't read disturbing stories, or watch horror movies on television. Quiet your mind and try to think about pleasant things as you wind down.

Lower the lights. The last hour or so before you turn in, dim the lights in your house. Bright light is a trigger for your internal clock to say, "Wake up!" But darkness brings on sleep.

Take a warm bath. It may get you ready for dreamland and help you sleep deeper as well.

Reserve the bed for sleep and sex. Don't eat, drink, read, or watch television in bed.

Practice gradual relaxation. While lying in bed, relax your muscles, starting with your toes. Continue relaxing each group of muscles, moving up your body. When you get to your scalp, all tension should be gone.

Don't stay in bed if you are not sleepy. If you are still awake after half an hour, get up and do some quiet activity. Go back to bed when you feel sleepy again.

Nature's checklist for a sound slumber

Sleeping pills may sometimes be appropriate for short-term use in times of stress or illness. But for a healthier choice without serious side effects, consider these natural sleep aids.

Valerian is a valuable herb that has been used for centuries as a mild sedative. In recent studies, those who took valerian reported that they got to sleep faster and slept better. In the U.S., you can find capsules containing 400-530 mg whole ground valerian root. They are generally taken 30 to 60 minutes before bedtime.

You may also find capsules of a root extract, liquid extracts, and tinctures. And you can make a tea of the dried root, using one teaspoon per cup.

Valerian is on the list of herbs generally considered safe by the Food and Drug Administration (FDA). It is sometimes used to treat uterine contractions, so if you are pregnant, check with your doctor before using this herb.

Lavender has a sweet scent that slips you into slumber. Just taking a deep breath can be relaxing. When that breath brings with it a pleasant smell, it's even more soothing.

British researchers discovered that some elderly people were able to give up sleeping pills when the scent of lavender filled their bedrooms. They rested better, and their normal sleep patterns returned without the side effects of sleep medications.

This finding could provide a "scent-sational" alternative to the tranquilizers and drugs that are usually prescribed for insomnia.

Melatonin is a natural hormone produced in the pineal gland that lies at the base of your brain. It brings on a desire to sleep in darkness and triggers alertness in daylight.

Some studies show that taking artificial melatonin supplements may help bring on sleep. It seems to help night workers shift their sleep cycle as well as help travelers avoid jet lag. Although you can find melatonin supplements in your health food store, it's still in the experimental stages and is not regulated by the FDA.

Try increasing your melatonin levels naturally by eating oats, sweet corn, rice, ginger, tomatoes, bananas, and barley. Also:

- Keep your bedroom very dark.

- Get eight hours of sleep every night.

- Get plenty of sunshine during the day.

13 kinds of sleep-defeating drugs

The next time you reach for a pill to help you sleep, take a look at the other drugs in your medicine cabinet. One of them may hold the answer to your sleepless nights.

Several types of drugs can cause insomnia as a side effect. Some of the most common are:

- antihypertensives
- beta-blockers
- decongestants
- levodopa
- phenytoin (Dilantin)
- theophylline
- antineoplastics
- corticosteroids
- diuretics
- oral contraceptives
- stimulants
- thyroid hormone
- selective serotonin reuptake inhibitors and protriptyline (Vivactil)

If you suspect a drug you are taking is interfering with your sleep, talk with your doctor about switching to another medication or lowering the dosage. Don't stop taking the drug without his approval.

It's also a good idea to read the labels on any over-the-counter drugs you're taking. Look for alcohol or caffeine in the ingredients list. These sleep-busters could be keeping you awake.

Sleep together, sleep better

Are you losing sleep over whether or not to get married or quit your job? You might put your mind and body to rest by doing one or both.

Married people and those who don't work full time tend to get more sleep than single folks and those employed full time. That's what researchers found when they studied young adults between 26 and 35 years old at a sleep disorders clinic in Michigan.

Those who were married reported much less sleepiness during the day. Researchers believe they follow a lifestyle with more orderly patterns than their less-settled single peers. And those who work full time have less opportunity to take naps to catch up on some of the sleep lost due to a busy night life.

If you are married, snuggle up and enjoy pleasant dreams, even if you have to get up and go to work in the morning. At least you'll face the day well-rested.

Beware of sleep 'overdose'

Just as you can overeat, you can also sleep too much. Rather than feeling rested afterwards, you wind up tired and grumpy. Excessive slumber can also have more serious results. You are more at risk of stroke or heart disease if you sleep more than eight hours a day or take naps during the day. And doing both puts you at even greater risk for these problems.

Believe it or not, a short night's sleep may bring the lift you need when you feel down. It's not understood just why, but people who are clinically depressed are sleepier but happier when they get only four hours of sleep. Their lighter mood wears off, however, after returning to a normal night's sleep.

If you think you sleep too much, you might experiment with a shorter night. And don't take naps — you may feel more rested without them. With the extra time, you can keep up your spirits with a new hobby or spending time with old friends.

"Men and gods alike bow to sleep in submission."

— Homer, The Illiad

How to escape serious sleep loss

Many people with sleep disorders don't realize their problem is serious enough to need treatment. But these problems can worsen if ignored. And they may be symptoms of other illnesses. Each of the following requires a different treatment. If you suspect you have one, see your doctor or a sleep specialist.

Insomnia is the most common sleep disorder. If it doesn't last long, or comes and goes, you can usually handle it with a few habit changes. But if sleeplessness is a problem almost every night and continues for a month or more, you have chronic insomnia. This is more serious and may lead to irritability, fatigue, and other health problems. It also increases your chances of a psychiatric disability such as depression, anxiety, or alcohol problems.

Follow the tips given throughout this chapter to help relieve your insomnia. If it becomes chronic, see your doctor for a thorough evaluation.

Restless leg syndrome can keep you tossing and turning. You may experience uncomfortable sensations in the foot, calf, or upper legs.

It's usually most bothersome late in the day or in the evening, mainly when you are at rest. It is especially noticeable when you first lie down and are trying to fall asleep.

To relieve the sensations, rub, stretch, or bend your legs, or get up and walk around. Although bothersome, it's generally harmless and may come and go over the years.

Narcolepsy affects the part of the central nervous system that controls sleep and wakefulness. Watch out for these symptoms:

- You fall asleep at an inappropriate time such as while eating or talking.

- You experience a sudden loss of muscle tone.

- You find you can't move when falling asleep or waking up.

- You have unpleasant dream-like experiences as you are dozing off.

- You waken frequently during the night.

- You experience memory and learning difficulties.

If you notice these symptoms, you should avoid driving or operating heavy machinery. Your doctor can advise you on the best way to relieve this serious condition.

Sleep apnea can leave you gasping for breath during the night because of a severe lack of oxygen. This is a potentially life-threatening disorder that may also lead to heart attack or stroke.

Your sleeping partner may be more apt than you to notice some of the symptoms. You may not remember that you snorted or gasped frequently during the night. You may, however, be aware of how sleepy you feel the next day. You may be irritable and depressed, lose interest in sex, or have headaches. You may also notice problems with memory and learning.

Some ways to help this problem:

- **Try not to sleep on your back.** Sew a tennis or ping pong ball into a pocket on the back of your pajamas so you'll be forced to sleep on your side.

- **Reduce stress.** By lowering your anxiety or depression, you improve your chances for a deeper sleep. Try some gentle stretching and deep-breathing exercises before bedtime, focusing on a routine that will calm and relax you.

- **Lose weight.** Statistics show this problem is more common if you're overweight.

- **Guard your mouth.** A properly fitted mouth guard, worn while sleeping, can reposition your tongue and jaw so your throat stays open.

- **Mask it.** A new treatment for sleep apnea forces your airway to stay open by blowing air from a compressor into a face mask you wear over your nose and mouth.

- **Seek surgery.** This is probably the only course that will cure sleep apnea.

Parasomnias are abnormal events that occur during the deepest part of your sleep cycle. Here are some suggestions on how to deal with the most typical ones.

- **Sleep walking** is common in children and tends to run in families. An episode may last a few minutes or an hour, but the chances are good you won't remember it. Although sleepwalkers tend to maneuver safely most of the time, there is danger of falling or wandering outside. Take steps to secure your sleeping area with locks on outside doors and gates at the head and foot of stairs. And clear the sleeping area of dangerous objects like knives.

- **Sleep talking** is harmless but may be irritating to a sleeping partner. It can be brought on by stress or illness or may be associated with sleep apnea. Fortunately, it is usually temporary. Taking steps to deal with the underlying cause should eliminate the problem.

- **Sleep eating** may occur in association with sleep walking, sleep apnea, or restless leg syndrome. It can also result from medications prescribed for depression or insomnia. The sleeper may not be aware of the nightly visits to the refrigerator or pantry. Since there is danger of weight gain, choking, or injury from a cut or burn while preparing food, you might want to use a lock on the kitchen door.

Wired for sleep

If you think you have a serious sleep disorder, see your doctor. After he checks you out, he might suggest you spend a night or two in a sleep clinic. What goes on there may seem quite mysterious. But knowing what to expect can reduce any anxiety you may have.

You've probably seen pictures of people in these clinics. They look like they have wires coming out of their heads. Actually these wires are connected to electrodes that are attached to the outside of your scalp. They measure your brain activity.

Doctors record your breathing, heart rate, muscle activity, and other body functions. A sleep technician may watch and make notes, or a camera may videotape your movements during sleep.

You may think it would be impossible to sleep in a strange place, hooked up to odd machines, with strangers watching you. But most people find they settle in pretty quickly and fall asleep with the same ease or difficulty they experience at home.

Just knowing that sleep experts can help you find ways to get more rest may be all you need to relax.

Tips for beating the shift-work blues

If you work a non-traditional shift, it may be even harder to keep your body rested and your thinking sharp. Neither your mind nor your body adjusts easily to working at night and sleeping during the day. But you can help yourself get a more restful sleep. Start with the tips already mentioned and add these:

- Darken your room as much as possible with shades, blinds, or draperies. Or wear an eye mask. Unplug the phone and consider using ear plugs, or run a fan to block out noise.

- If you prefer to sleep right after the night shift, avoid morning sunlight as much as possible while driving home. Sunlight has a powerful effect on your biological clock, making you more alert. If it's still dark, head straight home. If it's already light, wear wrap-around sunglasses.

- On weekends, stick to your usual sleep schedule. If you have to change shifts, try adjusting your sleeping time an hour or two each day to help you ease into the new schedule.

Sleeping well during your off hours helps you stay more alert on the job and healthier in the long run. Without enough sleep, you're more at risk for work-related accidents as well as problems at home. Do yourself and your family a favor and put sleep first on your daily "to do" list.

It pays to sleep on the job

Grabbing 40 winks at work once might have gotten you fired. Today your employer may see it as a sign of your interest in safety and productivity. Believe it or not, naps are becoming more acceptable for grown-ups, even in the workplace.

Your body most likely wants to sleep from 2 a.m. to 4 a.m. and the same hours in the afternoon. Slugging down a lot of coffee may have been your way of making it through one of these slow periods. But a nap is more natural, more refreshing, and may leave you more alert afterwards.

So don't be surprised if your boss suggests you put your head on your desk for 20 to 30 minutes. Some companies are even creating rooms with beds or cots for napping.

Sleep experts warn, however, that too long a nap is not a good idea. More than 40 minutes and you may find it hard to wake up, leaving you drowsy and less productive.

Helpful hints for tired travelers

Driving can sometimes be monotonous and boring. Your brain can slow down, making it hard to stay alert. Some safety experts think drowsy drivers may now cause more accidents than drunk drivers. But you can prevent sleep-related accidents if you think ahead.

- Don't drive when you are sleepy, taking medications that cause drowsiness, or drinking alcohol. You are most likely to be sleepy between midnight and 6 a.m. On long trips, stop to rest about every 100 miles or every two hours. And share the driving with a companion, if possible.

- Watch out for signs of mental fatigue. You probably sense when you are getting sluggish, but don't count on those feelings alone. Ask yourself if you can remember the last few miles. Are you yawning repeatedly and struggling to keep your eyes open and head up? Do you find yourself drifting out of your lane, tailgating, or missing traffic signs? Any of these can mean you are too sleepy to continue driving. As a temporary measure, drink a caffeinated beverage while finding a safe place to stop.

- Some people find that sniffing the aroma of peppermint oil helps them stay awake. Research has found that peppermint may have a positive effect when you're most sleepy.

- You may think that playing the radio or opening the window makes you more alert, but these measures are not helpful for long. Unless you have a rested driver who can take over for you, stop and take a 20- to 40-minute nap instead.

- Technology, in the form of a battery-operated alertness monitor, is coming to the rescue of some sleepy drivers. This device, which attaches to glasses, watches your eyes for signs that you are sleepy, then sounds an alarm. For more information on this device, contact MTI Research Inc., 7 Littleton Road, Westford, MA 01886.

Easy way to let the air out of jet lag

When you travel by air, falling asleep isn't a problem — unless you're the pilot. But if you cross multiple time zones, your sleep difficulties are likely to start after you arrive at your destination. That's when your body's biological clock may struggle with the different day/night cycle. As a result, you may experience insomnia, poor concentration, fatigue, irritability, loss of appetite, and diarrhea. To adjust quickly and be at your best, follow these tips.

Change your schedule. A few days before leaving on your trip, start adjusting your sleep schedule. The goal is to go to bed an hour earlier or later for each time zone crossed, depending on the direction you're going.

Time your arrival. Take a flight that arrives in early evening and stay up until 10 p.m. local time. Set your alarm clock to your regular wake-up time.

Stay awake during the day. You'll adjust faster if you stay awake all day. But if you really need a nap, don't sleep longer than two hours.

Dine when the locals do. Getting your body on the local time schedule is the key. Eating at about the same time as everyone else will help.

Eat small meals. When your body is trying to adjust to a new schedule, don't make it work hard by digesting a lot of food. For the first day or two, keep away from the buffet and have light meals instead.

Skip the caffeine and alcohol. Avoid caffeine and alcohol right before bedtime. They can interfere with your sleep.

Keep moving. You'll sleep better at night if you get some exercise during the day, but avoid strenuous activity right before bedtime.

Soak up some sun. Spending time outside in natural daylight will help readjust your internal clock.

Drink up. Don't take a chance on becoming dehydrated, especially if you've traveled to a higher elevation. Make sure you drink plenty of fluids.

Try melatonin. Melatonin supplements may help fight the effects of jet lag. In one study, people who traveled across eight time zones had less jet lag if they took 5 milligrams (mg) of melatonin daily, starting three days before they left home. For ways to increase melatonin naturally, see *Nature's checklist for a sound slumber*.

Spring forward safely

With springtime comes daylight savings time and an extra hour you can spend outside at the end of the day. You may enjoy planting flowers, tossing a Frisbee, or just catching up on neighborhood news.

Unfortunately, this bright picture has a dark side. During the first few days of daylight savings time, you are more likely to have a traffic accident. A Canadian study reported in *The New England Journal of Medicine* found about 8 percent more traffic accidents on the first Monday after the spring time change. Drivers were less alert because they lost one hour of sleep.

Avoiding this problem seems simple enough. On the night when daylight savings time goes into effect, just go to bed an hour earlier and wake up an hour earlier. Same amount of sleep, right?

Sadly, it just doesn't work that smoothly. Researchers say it takes about five days for your body clock to fully adjust to the time change.

The best way to prepare for a safe "spring forward" is to ease forward. Start adjusting your sleep time a week before the start of daylight savings time. Set your alarm clock for 10 minutes earlier each morning and go to bed 10 minutes earlier each night. Your body clock should accept this gradual adjustment more readily.

Fortunately, when fall comes, researchers find a drop in accidents equal to the increase in spring.

Wacky ways to fall asleep

If you are really desperate for a peaceful snooze and haven't found anything that helps, you might try a few of these unusual ideas. They may seem weird, but at least one person out there swears by each of them.

- Sleep with a pillow over your head but not over your face.

- Wear a hat to bed. (This person may have gotten the idea from the children's book, *Miss Twiggley's Tree*. Funny Miss Twiggley lived in a tree and slept in her hat.)

- Read something really boring like a psychological journal article.

- Imagine you are a cat and stretch like one. Extend your legs and arms as far as possible for about 15 minutes. Purr if the mood strikes you.

- Sleep in a cold room. In summer, turn the air down to about 60 degrees. If you let the cold air hit your feet, you may cool down faster. In the winter, leave your bedroom windows open about one to two inches to let the cold air in.

- Imagine driving down a highway. Pretend you see a billboard ahead with the word "SLEEP" on it.

- Sniff some chopped onion. Keep it in a jar beside your bed. Open it and smell it at bedtime. You should be asleep in 15 minutes.

- Give yourself a stomach massage. Start at your navel and make gentle circles with your hand in a clockwise direction. Make your circles bigger and bigger until you reach the outside of your stomach. Then make gradually smaller circles going back to the navel. Do it again in a counter-clockwise direction. Repeat the whole process with the other hand. If you fall asleep and forget where you were, you've succeeded.

- Try gently rocking your body like you would rock a baby while sitting in a straight chair, not a rocking chair. The motion is from side to side rather than back and forth. You may find it pretty relaxing.

- Get someone to pay you to sleep. In a study at a sleep center in England, people who were paid money actually fell asleep faster.

- Visualize the details of a peaceful, calming scene. When you've really got it clear in your mind, imagine a comfortable spot to lie down. Curl up and go to sleep.

- If all else fails, go back to the old stand-by — counting sheep, old sweethearts, the number of cars you hear passing, your breaths — anything that will bore you into sleep.

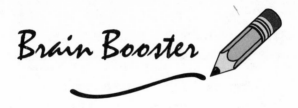

Bedtime logic problem

Last night on the television talk show *Nightlight*, host Dan Rouser interviewed celebrities about their sleep habits. The five guests included three stage entertainers (a singer, a dancer, and an actor), a popular politician, and a medal-winning ice skater.

All admitted their schedules sometimes make it difficult to get a good night's sleep, but each had a different preferred bedtime for when they weren't working or training. (The earliest was 10:30 p.m.)

Rouser found that all five celebrities enjoyed sleeping in flannel pajamas but liked different patterns. One preferred a wild animal print, while another chose a tartan plaid.

From the clues on the following page, can you tell the name (one is Dozzer), profession, preferred bedtime, and favorite pajamas of each guest on the show?

Check your answers in the *Solutions to Brain boosters and teasers* section at the back of the book.

1. The three stage entertainers like bedtimes that come one directly after the other in this order: actor, singer, and dancer.

2. Napper (who wears polka dot pajamas) likes to go to bed sometime later than the one who sleeps in plaid pajamas and immediately before the politician (who doesn't wear teddy bears.)

3. The actor prefers to go to bed earlier than the celebrity who sleeps in plaid.

4. If Nodder goes to bed at 11:30, then he is the dancer. Otherwise, he is the ice skater (who goes to bed immediately after the one who wears wild animal print pajamas).

5. Dozzer goes to bed before the singer.

6. Shuteye likes to turn in sometime after the one who likes striped pajamas but sometime before the dancer.

Answer chart:

Name	Profession	Pajamas	Bedtime

Instructions: Use this chart to help you find the solutions based on what you learn from the clues. Put an "X" for "no" and an "O" for "yes." When you record a "yes" (O), the rest of the same line and column in the section where it is placed must be a "no" (X).

	Profession					Pajama pattern					Bedtime				
	Actor	Dancer	Ice skater	Politician	Singer	Candy stripes	Polka dots	Tartan plaid	Teddy bears	Wild animals	10:30	11:00	11:30	12:30	1:00
Knight															
Dozzer															
Napper															
Nodder															
Shuteye															
10:30															
11:00															
11:30															
12:30															
1:00															
Bears															
Stripes															
Plaid															
Polka dots															
Wild animals															

Dreaming

Your brain takes a 'working' vacation

You arrive at your new boss's townhouse on a dark, cold winter's day. His young wife, wearing a bathing suit, meets you at the door. You recognize her as the sister of a boyhood friend. You see your boss approaching and extend your hand in greeting.

Suddenly he becomes your fifth grade history teacher. You are now seated in a desk much too small for you. Your old friend's sister, wearing a long white wedding gown, is standing at the classroom door asking angrily why you left her at your boss's house alone. You take her by the hand and fly with her over the neighborhood where you lived as a child.

If you were having this dream, it would be as real to you as anything you do when you are wide awake. But in the light of day your dream world seems like a crazy mixed-up place where things happen with no rhyme or reason.

Could these dreams mean anything? Ancient people thought so. They searched them for divine signs and prophecies as well as simple guidance in their daily lives. The Bible tells how a dream's warning sent Joseph and Mary into hiding with the infant Jesus.

And some native cultures think that dreams aren't in your mind at all. They believe you actually travel to a parallel world that's just as real as the one you live in while awake.

Your dreams may contain amazing stories that delight and entertain you or terrifying nightmares that disturb your peace of mind. But as far as your brain is concerned, whatever they mean, your dreams are critical to your health and well being.

> *"Dreaming is like being transported to another world*
> *— at the speed of thought!"*
>
> — Cohen

Energize your day with the right kind of sleep

Do you have fun sharing your dreams with your family at the breakfast table? If so, you are getting good REM sleep each night. REM stands for rapid eye movement because your eyes dart from side to side when you are having this kind of sleep.

Sleep scientists say that everybody dreams while they are in REM. You may think you don't, but if somebody wakes you at the right time, you'll probably remember one.

And not only does REM sleep give you dreams, it also helps you wake up in a better mood. In sleep laboratories, when people are continually awakened during REM sleep, they are more irritable the next day. Those whose non-REM sleep gets disturbed may wake up sleepier but not grumpier.

It's not clear if it's the dreams or some other aspect of REM sleep that's important, but experts say you need it. The brain seems to agree. If you don't get enough one night, it makes up for the loss by spending more time in REM the next night.

So how can you get more of this dream-filled sleep every night? Just sleep a little longer. REM comes and goes in a cycle that repeats about every 90 minutes. In the first cycle of the night it lasts only five to 10 minutes, but it gets longer with each cycle. If you sleep seven or more hours, your last 45 to 60 minutes may be all REM. If you sleep six hours or less, you miss out on the best dream time.

The last dreams of the night are the most intense. During this time your brain may be working harder than it does when you are awake. Non-REM sleep is more restful sleep. But REM sleep gets the credit if you wake up feeling happy and with a dream or two worth sharing.

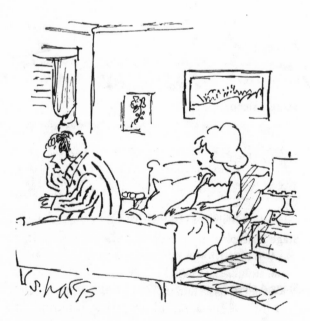

Boy are my eyes tired! I had REM sleep all night long.

How to REMember your dreams

Do you have trouble remembering your dreams? Most of us do, but if you really want to, you can learn how to capture those hard-to-hold fantasies.

Start by getting a full night's sleep. Remember, the most vivid dreams usually come during the last part of your sleep. Follow these practices every night, and you will probably begin to remember them.

Keep a dream journal by your bed. Before going to bed, write down whatever has been on your mind that day and the kinds of things you'd like to dream about. Then write the date and "Dream #1." This makes it clear to your subconscious that you expect to dream.

If you prefer, you can use a tape recorder. Then you won't need a light when you wake in the dark. You can also buy a pen with a small light, which is handy if you have a sleep partner you don't want to disturb.

Make your intent clear. Say to yourself firmly but gently as you are falling asleep, "I will remember my dreams." Repeat this a few times. But don't push. Keep a lighthearted, welcoming attitude about it.

Lie quietly and remember. When you wake after a dream, ask yourself what was going through your mind. Patiently allow images and bits and pieces of the dream to come to mind.

Write it down. If you wait until morning, you'll probably lose it. Include whatever fragments you recall. Note the emotions or sensations you feel. Later you can write any connections you think it might have to events from the past or issues you are concerned about. Write "Dream #2" in your journal to affirm your intent to remember another dream.

Avoid using an alarm clock. The dreams you have just before you wake up in the morning will usually be the longest and most intense. You are likely to lose them, however, if you suddenly wake up to the loud ringing of an alarm clock. And try not to let thoughts of the day ahead intrude until you have reviewed your dreams and recorded them.

Take note of your daydreams. Daytime fantasies are similar to nighttime dreams. So write and reflect on those as well.

Be patient. If you don't usually remember your dreams, it may take a few nights before you begin to recall them. And most people go through periods from time to time when they don't remember any.

Continue to invite them and they should return shortly. But don't be surprised if you have trouble remembering dreams during times of fatigue, stress, or emotional distress. Alcohol and drugs can also make them harder to remember.

"As my awareness increases,
my control over my own being increases."

— Will Schutz

Tap the power of your fantasy world

Now that you've learned how to remember your dreams, you can use them to make your life better. Some folks think dreams are just plain nonsense and best forgotten. Others brush them aside, saying, "It's *just* a dream." But your dreams can be like a counselor that's available to you every night.

Dreams help your brain sort through and organize what it has taken in during the day. Your earliest dreams of the night usually relate to ordinary events like what you did at work or a conversation you had with a friend. They may go back as far as the previous six to eight days.

These early dreams may also be a way to forget. It's like emptying the trash. There's no need to clutter your mind with the memory of every moment of every day. You want to store only what's important in your long-term memory.

As the night goes on, your dreams get richer in detail and plot. They are more emotional in tone and more often about your early childhood. These are the dreams you are most likely to remember and to learn from. But they may not be sweet dreams. Research shows that overall, more dreams are negative or unpleasant than they are positive.

If this is true, why then, would you want to remember them? Dream researcher Robert Van de Castle poses this question in his book, *Our Dreaming Mind*. His response is that if you pay attention to those troublesome dreams, you have a better chance of reducing stress and anxiety in your waking life. He says your dreams tell you about things that need your attention and give you clues about what you can do to make things better.

Van de Castle thinks that checking up on your emotional health through your dreams is like seeing your doctor for a physical examination. You might catch problems before they become serious or get the encouraging news that you are in great shape. Best of all, you don't have to make an appointment with your dreams, and they don't send you a bill! You just have to pay attention to them, and they'll give you valuable information for free.

Unlock the secrets of your nighttime visions

Your dreams have messages just for you. Even if someone else had the same dream as yours, chances are the meaning would be quite different. The language of dreams is symbols and metaphors. That means the things that appear in your dreams will usually stand for something else.

Dream messages aren't always easy to see right away, so you'll need patience and commitment. But if you are willing to work at it, you can understand your dreams and learn from them.

The more information you get about dream interpretation and the more you practice, the easier it will be to find the methods that work best for you. You'll find it helpful to read books by respected dream experts like Robert Van de Castle, Gayle Delaney, and Jeremy Taylor. Meanwhile, these tips will help you get started with your dream study.

Give your dream a title. Think of a few words that describe the story of your dream. Write the title at the top of the entry in your dream journal. Make it brief but clear, like "Searching for my father's lost bankbook."

Consider the emotions you felt in your dream. When do these same emotions occur in your life? Are they connected to something you have been concerned about recently?

Make associations to people and things in your life. If you dream of a friend, ask yourself what words come to mind when you think of her. Is she talkative and outgoing, often the center of attention? What part of yourself would like to have your attention, to be acknowledged? Think of every possible connection.

Pay attention to the feeling of "Ah ha!" Notice when something pops into your mind that really feels right to you. The chances are good you are on the right track to understanding the meaning of your dream.

Go back into the dream. Sometimes you will wake up before you finish a dream. You may feel the need to complete it in order to understand it. Return to the dream by relaxing, closing your eyes and recalling the dream. When you reach the point at which you woke up, continue imagining how the dream might have unfolded. You can also go back into a completed dream for more information.

Hold a conversation with a dream character. This imaginary discussion can work with an object from your dream as well as a character. The drab-looking bridge you saw just briefly might have a lot to tell you. Maybe it's tired of bearing the burden of people walking on it. Does it bring to your attention some way you are letting others take advantage of you? Perhaps it's time to talk to family members about more help with household duties.

Of course, the bridge might say how strong and important it feels supporting so many cars as they cross the river. But it would enjoy a new paint job. (Have you thought about asking for a nicer office since you got that promotion to a more responsible position?)

Draw sketches of dream images. A picture, so they say, is worth a thousand words. Sometimes you can see additional details in what you draw. You don't have to be a talented artist. Even stick figures might reveal something meaningful you missed in recalling and writing about your dream.

Notice patterns in your dreams. From time to time go back and read through the titles or even entire dreams. The themes that keep repeating can give you an idea of what you still haven't resolved. Topics that don't come up anymore may show how you've changed since you started working with your dreams.

During times of distress you may want to get help with understanding your dream messages. A professional who works with dreams can provide support and a safe environment for dealing with deeper emotions. But remember there is always more than one possible meaning for any dream, and you are the final authority on yours.

> *"Dreaming is an act of pure imagination,*
> *attesting in all men a creative power,*
> *which, if it were available in waking,*
> *would make every man a Dante or a Shakespeare."*
>
> — H.F. Hodges

Problem solving in your sleep

Professional golfer Jack Nicklaus was struggling with a bad slump. Then one night he dreamed of holding his golf club in a different way and making a perfect swing. When he tried it the next day, it worked just as it had in the dream. With his new grip, he was able to shoot back into a successful career.

Mohandas Gandhi was looking for a nonviolent way to help free the people of India from Great Britain's rule. He dreamed the idea of a nation-wide 24-hour fast. It worked in bringing the people together. It got the attention of the British and helped gain India's independence.

Harriet Tubman was a brave woman who helped runaway slaves reach freedom. She said her dreams helped her find safe escape routes. With their help she never lost a "passenger" on the "Underground Railroad."

Hatch an answer to your dilemma. A hen knows what to do after she lays an egg. She patiently sits on it, expecting it to hatch a baby chick. You can "hatch" a dream solution to a problem by preparing your mind for answers, then sleeping on it. This process is called "incubating" a dream.

Choose a situation that is causing a problem. Think about it before you fall asleep. Go over any solutions you have considered. Don't agonize over it. Just calmly think it through.

Decide what you might like your dream to do. Do you want a dream that shows the best of two choices you are considering? Do you need additional information before making a decision? Maybe you would like some insights about what is causing the problem.

In your dream journal go ahead and write a title related to the goal of this dream. For example, "How I can get along better with my boss," or "Finding money to repair my car." As you fall asleep, gently repeat a statement of what you expect from your dream. ("My dream will tell me where to get money to pay for my car repairs.")

When you record your dreams, be open to messages that might surprise you. Your dreaming mind may have ideas you hadn't considered. And pay close attention to the way your dreams end. Often the last part of the dream gives the best clues to solving your problems. If you wake up before the dream ends, lie quietly recalling the dream. Imagine how the dream might have ended.

If you don't get an answer the first night, try again the next. Don't push, but don't give up too quickly either. You'll probably get help if you stay with the process.

Learn from lucid dreams. Some people can tell they are in the midst of a dream while it's going on. This is called lucid dreaming. Most of the time when people first have lucid dreams they wake up as soon as they realize it. Others have more control over these dreams. They can choose to wake up if it's unpleasant. Or they can decide the direction they want the dream to go. It's somewhat like writing the script for a play.

Jeremy Taylor, in *Where People Fly and Water Runs Uphill*, tells the story of how a man he calls Alex used a lucid dream to break his heavy smoking habit. Alex dreamed of being chased by a fire-breathing dragon. As he was running away in fear, he suddenly realized he was dreaming. He stopped in his tracks and turned to face the dragon. He demanded to know why it was chasing him and frightening him so.

The dragon responded that he was Alex's smoking addiction.

As he looked more closely, Alex could see a disgusting brown, sticky slime oozing out of the dragon's body. Its rancid smell was sickening. He shouted to the dragon to get away from him. He no longer wanted this repulsive creature in his life.

On awakening, Alex found he no longer wanted to smoke.

Dream expert Dr. Stephen LaBerge believes most people, if they really want to, can have lucid dreams. He and his associates at the Lucidity Institute in Palo Alto, California, teach people how. They suggest you practice recalling your dreams until you are remembering at least one each night.

Then they suggest you identify "dreamsigns." This is what LaBerge calls anything in your dream that lets you know you are dreaming. (Things that couldn't happen in your waking life, like driving a car across the surface of a lake.)

To get in the habit of noticing the difference between dreams and awake-time, LaBerge recommends a reality-testing technique. He suggests you practice this several times a day. Maybe choose certain times you'll do it — every time you look in the mirror, look at your watch, or arrive home from work. The more often the better.

- Carry something with you that has words or numbers that don't change, like a business card or a non-digital watch. As a reality test, look at the words or numbers. Look away, then look back again. Ask yourself if they changed. Try to make them change while looking at them. If you are awake, they won't change; but if you were dreaming, they might.

- Remind yourself that you aren't dreaming now. But ask yourself, if you were dreaming, how things might change. Try to use all your senses to visualize dream-like images and scenes. Imagine doing things possible only in dreams, like floating off the ground.

- Imagine yourself doing something you'd enjoy doing in a dream. For example, you might like to jump over trees or ride a bicycle up the side of a building.

When you are ready to go to sleep, follow the technique LaBerge calls MILD (mnemonic induction of lucid dreams).

- In the relaxed state just before falling asleep, tell yourself that you will wake up when you have a dream. When you do wake up, recall as much detail of the dream as possible.

- Returning to sleep again, tell yourself sincerely, "The next time I dream, I will remember I am dreaming." Continue to focus on this one thought.

- Imagine you are back in the dream you just woke from and that you realize it is a dream. Watch for a dreamsign, something that wouldn't be there if you were awake. If you didn't remember a dream when you woke up, imagine being in one you had recently. When you see a dreamsign, say to yourself, "I'm dreaming." Imagine doing whatever you had decided you'd like to do in your lucid dream, like jumping over the trees.

- Repeat this process until you fall asleep. If other thoughts intrude, go back to this process so that it's the last thing that happens before you fall asleep.

Lucid dreaming, especially when combined with dream incubation, might help you change bad habits, improve your tennis serve, or have more peaceful relationships. But some people like lucid dreams for the pure adventure of them.

Dr. Gayle Delaney is a therapist who helps people explore meanings of their dreams. She has written several books, including *In Your Dreams*, a guide to understanding the most common dreams — like those about falling.

Does falling occur more often in a "bad" dream? Yes, according to Dr. Delaney. But sometimes it can be turned into something positive.

"I can't recall a positive falling dream except for reports of lucid ones in which a dreamer begins to fly and is relieved or amused and delighted by the flight," she says. "But the falling part always seems to be scary."

If you are afraid of falling dreams, maybe you can turn them into fun. Practice your lucid dreaming, then put on your superman pajamas and fly happily above the clouds.

Learn Spanish in your sleep? Dream on

Have you ever dreamed of a fire drill or of someone ringing your door bell and on awakening realized the telephone was ringing? Your brain can take the sounds you hear while you sleep and use it in your dreams.

So you may wonder if you can learn math or a foreign language by playing a taped lesson while you sleep. Students everywhere wish it were that simple. Unfortunately, research shows this just doesn't happen.

The advertisements for those learn-while-you sleep products can be quite convincing. But the truth is, you forget most of what you hear even five minutes *before* you go to sleep.

But you can use sleep to learn better. Check out the *Sleep* chapter to find out how the right kind of slumber can help improve your learning skills.

Escape the menace of nightmares

You are walking alone down a dark street late at night. You hear footsteps behind you. As you walk faster, the footsteps follow at the same pace. Frightened now, you begin running. Breathlessly you reach your door and are fumbling with your keys when — you wake up, perspiring and with your heart pounding.

If you are like most people, at some time in your life you have awakened from a terrifying dream, filled with fear and anxiety. The chances are good you dreamed of being chased. That's the most common theme in nightmares.

What brings on your nightmares, and what can you do about them? Some nightmares are caused by illness or medication. Others are related to the stresses of a job or relationship, financial problems, pregnancy, or other daily life issues. And some people who are especially sensitive, emotional, and creative seem to have them for no reason at all.

Night terrors are not the same as nightmares. You are more likely to have one earlier in the night. You may be harder to awaken and likely will remember the terror but not much in the way of images or a dream story.

It's not clear what causes night terrors. Children who have them may also sleepwalk or wet the bed. They usually stop having them by the time they reach puberty. In adults they may be associated with stress. If they are particularly disturbing or frequent, you may want to see your doctor.

But don't despair about normal nightmares. Like other dreams, they are the perfect opportunity to explore the emotions that may relate to problems in your waking life.

A better ending. If you keep having the same disturbing dream, you might first want to work on reducing its power to frighten you. Then you can figure out its meaning.

Researchers have found that if you change the way the nightmare ends, you won't have it as often, and it will be less terrifying. Begin by recording it. Then rewrite it giving it a pleasing ending. For example, if someone is chasing you, you might imagine that as he gets closer he calls your name. You recognize the voice of a close friend. He wants to give you a gift. You stop and have a friendly chat.

Get in a comfortable position and relax. Close your eyes and imagine being in a safe, pleasant location. When you feel calm and peaceful, visualize the dream with its new ending. Repeat this process frequently until the nightmare no longer disturbs you.

The power of healing. If you suffer a severe accident, loss of a loved one, an assault, or other traumatic event, you may have nightmares for a while. This seems to be one way your mind helps you deal with the overwhelming emotions that follow. At first, the nightmare may be almost an exact replay of the incident. The feeling of terror may be nearly as strong as when it occurred.

But as time goes on, the "story" of the dream gradually changes. It includes new parts and drops some of the old scenes. The emotions are still similar but not as strong.

Frequently, there is a pattern of guilt in the dreams after trauma, especially if the victim survives and others do not. But as these dreams change they gradually get less intense.

In time they should no longer be disturbing. If they continue to upset you, however, you might want to consult a therapist.

An improved attitude. Not everybody who has bad dreams is particularly disturbed by them. Research shows that about half of the people who have frequent nightmares view them as interesting or brush them aside as "just dreams." If you can see them as dramatic opportunities to learn, you might even come to enjoy "riding" your nightmares.

Your fear may have something to do with your having frightening dreams in the first place. It's rare for nightmares to take place in a sleep laboratory. Sleepers there probably feel watched over and cared for. Children who wake after a bad dream usually don't have another in the same night if the parents take them into the safety of their bed.

Jeremy Taylor has studied dreams from a variety of perspectives for more than 25 years. He believes there is no such thing as a "bad" dream because even nightmares help you become healthy and whole.

Taylor says nightmares bring important messages in ways that are hard to ignore. They tell you to wake up and be aware of your feelings. So while they have your attention, why not let them teach you something that makes your life better?

Sleep with your 'doctor' for a diagnosis

We certainly aren't suggesting that you sleep with your human doctor (unless he's your mate), but your "dream doctor" can sometimes give you clues about an illness before you notice any symptoms. Dreams deal mainly with emotion. And if you are like most folks, you can get pretty emotional about your health.

Research shows that certain emotions come up more frequently in your dreams if you have a particular health condition. So paying attention to the mood of your dreams can give you a head start on prevention.

If, for example, you have a lot of anger and hostility in your dreams, you may want to have your blood pressure checked. Studies find that these two frequently go together.

But dreams, as you know, can have a lot of different meanings. So don't panic if you think you are getting a warning about your health. Think about all the possible interpretations. But if you get that "Ah ha" feeling when you consider an illness, it's a good idea to check it out with your doctor.

Dream messengers send clues to the future

Have you ever had a dream of an event that later happened just the way you dreamed it? If so, you had what is called a precognitive dream. The Bible tells of them, and so does history.

Samuel Clemens, who later became famous as the writer Mark Twain, is said to have had one about his brother. In his dream, he saw a metal coffin sitting on two chairs with the body of his brother Henry inside. On his brother's chest was a bouquet of white flowers with one red flower in the center.

A few days later, Henry died after a riverboat explosion. When Clemens went to the temporary morgue, he found his brother's body exactly as he had dreamed it.

Not everybody who studies dreams believes they can foretell the future. Proof is hard to come by. Some scientific studies have been done, but the outcomes have been varied. However, two of the most famous dream analysts, Sigmund Freud and Carl Jung, believed strongly in them.

Can these paranormal dreams be helpful? Researcher Dr. Louisa B. Rhine collected thousands of reports of precognitive dreams. She found 433 events that could have ended differently if the dreamer had acted. Of these, only about 30 percent made the effort to do something to change the outcome.

Researcher Ian Stevenson, a psychiatrist at the University of Virginia, collected 19 reports that he believed were credible of dreams that preceded and predicted the sinking of the "unsinkable" ship, Titanic. Could that tragedy have been prevented? No one knows, but if you have a dream that seems to foretell the future, you may want to pay close attention to it.

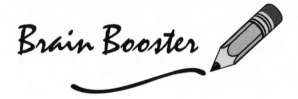

Fun facts dream quiz

How much dream trivia do you know? Answer these true-or-false questions, then check your knowledge in the *Solutions to Brain boosters and teasers* section at the back of the book.

1. Only mammals experience REM sleep.

2. Females dream about males more often than males dream about females.

3. If you dream you are falling and you hit the ground, you will die.

4. If you dream about a house with the roof falling in, it means you have a health problem, probably related to the head.

5. People who dream about flying are insecure.

6. Dreams have influenced great scientific thinkers, famous artists, and popular musicians.

7. Your birth order influences what you dream about.

8. Most dreams are in color.

9. Dreams often deal with reading, writing, and arithmetic.

10. Newborn babies spend more of their sleep time dreaming than adults.

Keeping your brain healthy

Your aging brain

How to keep your mind sharp

Charles Myers has a surprising request. He wants a computer. He wants to learn to "surf the net" and chat with other people his age. You probably don't think that's very surprising. These days, a computer is almost as common in households as televisions and telephones. But does it seem a little more unusual when you discover that Charles is 93 and recently moved to a nursing home? When he was born in 1904, computers weren't even dreamed of.

Most people would be surprised that a 93-year-old would want to learn about new technologies like computers. Some would doubt that he could. But "you can't teach an old dog new tricks" is one old saying that is just untrue.

Don't assume that because you're getting older, your brain will slow down. Take a lesson from Charles, and assume instead that you can do anything you set your mind to.

"When I was a boy of 14 my father was so ignorant
I could hardly stand to have the old man around.
But when I got to be 21, I was astonished
at how much he had learnt in seven years."

— Mark Twain

Reject aging-brain myths

As you get older, you may just accept the fact that time and the ravages of living take their toll on your brain, just as they do on other parts of your body. If arthritis and creaky knees are sure signs of an aging body, symptoms like senility, stroke, and Alzheimer's disease signal a similar decline in mind that many people expect as a normal part of aging.

However, you don't have to expect or accept such a decline. According to the most current research, your brain doesn't have to slow down as you age, and the mental problems that often seem to develop later in life can be prevented. In fact, if you were to examine two brains side by side, one belonging to a 25-year-old, and the other to a senior citizen of 75, it would be hard to see any physical differences between them.

It was once believed that you lost massive numbers of brain cells as you aged. Brain cells do shrink or die off gradually, beginning in young adulthood. By the time you are 80, your brain is about 5 percent smaller. But this is a small loss, which can be more than compensated for by increasing the connections between brain cells.

These connections between brain cells, synapses, provide communication pathways. Every time you learn something new, you build a new connection or strengthen an existing one. The more you learn as you age, the stronger your web of synapses becomes.

Some changes in mental abilities do occur as you get older. You may have some memory problems, but your ability to recognize information remains the same as younger people. If asked to recall meaningless information (nonsense syllables or unimportant events) the older you are, the more errors you make. If the material is meaningful, however, an older person's web of knowledge is more likely to catch it, so they show less decline in this area of mental ability.

It's never too late to bloom

Your brain is capable of great accomplishments, no matter what your age. Some people are late bloomers, while others begin early and continue to achieve for years. Grandma Moses didn't begin painting until she was in her late 70s, and she was still painting after age 100. Some other late achievers:

- Oliver Wendell Holmes remained on the Supreme Court until he was 90.

- Frank Lloyd Wright designed New York's Guggenheim Museum at age 89.

- Mary Baker Eddy founded the *Christian Science Monitor* at age 87.

- Phyllis Whitney published her 39th novel, *Amethyst Dreams*, at age 92.

- Benjamin Spock, famous baby doctor, was arrested at Cape Canaveral while demonstrating for world peace at age 83.

- George Bernard Shaw wrote several plays when he was in his 90s.

- Sidney Yates began his 15th term in the U.S. Congress at age 87.

- Kin Narita and Gin Kanie, Japanese twins, recorded a hit CD at the age of 99.

- Jacob Blitzstein graduated from high school at age 81.

Power up your mental strength with mental exercise

If your memory slips as you get older, you may automatically think Alzheimer's. But most memory problems in the elderly are caused by stress, depression, anxiety, too little sleep, and drug side effects, not Alzheimer's. Don't be alarmed because you misplace your glasses occasionally. That even happens to 21-year-olds. If you find your glasses and don't know what to do with them, however, you may have a problem.

In many ways, your brain is like any other part of your body — the more you take care of it, the better it will take care of you. And how do you take care of that glob of gray matter? That's right — just like any other part of your body. A good healthy diet, moderation in drinking, and sufficient sleep. Smoking is a no-no. Taking care of your brain now will help you avoid diseases associated with aging, like Alzheimer's. Of course, some factors that affect the aging of your brain are beyond your control — genetics for example.

But some researchers argue that, while all these factors are important, none are as critical as the one thing your brain absolutely needs to maintain its wit and wisdom — mental exercise.

Keep it constantly challenged. Recent medical studies have confirmed what many doctors have suspected for a long time. Your brain isn't fixed and unchangeable. Instead, it continues to grow and change as long as it is stimulated. When you keep your brain busy with new interests and challenges, it will respond by forming new electrical connections, adapting itself in response to what you feed it. In other words, not only can you maintain your mental sharpness as you get older, but you may actually get smarter.

About the best thing you can do for your brain is to keep it constantly challenged. Although not actually a muscle, of course, some scientists are convinced that your brain responds in much the same way. Work it, it grows. Let it lie, it starts to die. Just like your legs will grow weak if you never get out of your easy chair for a walk, your mind will not stay sharp if it is never given a reason to. Your brain requires continuous challenge to stay "in shape." If you want your thinker to perform like a champ, it's up to you to keep it in constant training.

Stretch its limits. Don't be nervous about exercising your brain. Keeping your brain challenged doesn't mean you have to spend your days reading encyclopedias and pondering the meaning of life. It is simply a matter of keeping your mind occupied, taking it off auto-pilot so that it has a daily chance to stretch its limits.

Suppose you take a walk every day for exercise. You've been doing it for years, usually walking at least a mile, and you feel like you're in pretty good shape. Then one day, you agree to help your sister move some boxes up from the basement to the attic. That night, to your surprise, your legs, knees, back, and neck are sore as can be. "What's this?" you say to yourself. "I'm in good shape; the mile I walk every day is a tougher workout than moving a few boxes."

This may be true, and you might be in fine shape. The problem is, you've varied your routine. Even if you use the same basic muscles to perform the task, you are forcing them to move in slightly different ways. Your soreness means your muscles have responded to the new challenge by stretching, expanding, and repairing themselves — in other words, growing.

The same principle applies to your mind, doctors say. Perhaps you have read the newspaper, balanced your finances, and talked to your interesting neighbor, the college professor, every day for years. That may seem like a good routine of mental exercise, but the problem lies in the routine. In order to give your bean a good workout, you need to vary your mental maneuvers. Stretch those far corners of your mind, wake up the thinking tools that thought they could get away with a nap. They won't get sore like your back, but they will get strong in new ways.

Below are some tips for keeping your mind on its toes:

Stay active. Leading a lifestyle that involves many activities gives you more opportunity to encounter new people, new situations, and new experiences to challenge your mind.

Be curious. Ask questions when you don't understand something. Some of the most powerful minds in history, such as Benjamin Franklin and Thomas Edison, were not necessarily more intelligent than others, but were certainly more curious.

Read. Perhaps the simplest and most available method for challenging your brain. Read many different types of material to maximize brain-building power.

Solve riddles. Puzzles, riddles, and mind games are excellent tools to stimulate your noggin. Challenges like crosswords and brain teasers force your mind to look at problems in new and unfamiliar ways.

Learn a new skill. Whether it's square dancing, calligraphy, or radio repair, the task of learning the skill is actually more important than the skill itself.

Finally, pick something you enjoy. What's the use of picking up a hobby that you will quickly abandon for lack of interest? Find a subject or a skill that seems interesting and challenging, and then set to it. Because, as with any other workout, the fitness of your brain depends mostly on your commitment to keep it up.

How to avoid brain-cell burnout

When it comes to brainpower, "use it or lose it" is great advice. Exercising your brain cells helps keep them healthy and builds new connections. The more of these connections you can build, the less likely you are to suffer mental diseases like Alzheimer's.

However, research finds that using the same brain cells for too long could cause them to burn out. Mental variety may be the key to keeping those brain cells healthy and alive. Exercise your brain cells, but switch activities frequently to prevent burn-out.

For example, working puzzles can give your brain healthy stimulation, so that's a great pastime. But varying the type of puzzles you do may spread the mental activity over a larger number of brain cells. Try crossword puzzles, jigsaw puzzles, *and* math puzzles.

Work out your body for a fitter brain

Mental exercise helps keep your brain young and healthy, but physical exercise benefits your brain too. Your daily walk or aerobics class may do more than keep your body youthful, fit, and ready for action. It may also keep your brain fit and ready to think.

Thinking is hard work. When you are concentrating on a problem, your brain cells need more nutrients and oxygen, which are provided through blood flow. Brain disorders associated with aging, like Alzheimer's disease, may be caused or aggravated by a decrease in blood flow to the brain.

However, a recent study found that rats that were physically active dramatically increased the new blood vessel growth in their brains. More blood vessels means more oxygen and nutrients feeding those hard-working brain cells. The increase took place within three days of beginning a wheel-treading exercise program.

The really good news about this study is that it used middle-aged rats. So if the findings translate to humans, even if you've been a couch potato all your life, you can still improve your brain by moving your muscles.

Old age at 25?

Taking care of your brain is more critical today because you'll probably use it much longer than your parents and grandparents did. The average life span has increased dramatically in the last few centuries.

- People in 1797 lived an average of only 25 years.

- A hundred years later, in 1897, life span had almost doubled to 48 years.

- In 1947, people lived an average of 65 years.

- In 1997, average life span had increased to 76.1 years.

- By 2027, you might expect to reach 100 years of age, and people living to 120 may not even be that unusual.

Attitude helps you remain ageless

Your great-uncle Fred is 101 and still works in his garden. Your neighbor down the street is 98, but she walks briskly past your house every day. What do these people have in common that keeps them young and healthy? Research finds that attitude may be the most important factor in remaining healthy well into your twilight years.

A recent study of people in their 80s and 90s found that sheer will-power may offset some of the physical decline you experience in later years. The people were interviewed about their ability to do daily tasks, their own impression of their health, and their sense of control over their lives.

The interviews revealed that people who function best and remain mobile as they get older have several traits in common.

- They believed they were healthy.

- They lived independently.

- They had a sense of mastery over their situation.

Researchers say that determination to remain independent gives some elders an edge over others their age.

Another study tracked Harvard graduates for more than 40 years and found that those who had the most pessimistic outlook at age 25 were struck by the most serious illnesses in their 60s.

Researchers believe negative attitudes like pessimism and a help-less outlook shorten your life by reducing your immune system's ability to fight off disease. The culprit in the attitude war is stress, which may be more damaging to your mind than anything.

A positive attitude and a sense of control can go a long way toward a long, healthy life. So decide what is most important to you, take charge, and believe you will succeed. You may add years to your life.

"In youth we learn; in age we understand."
— Marie von Ebner-Eschenbach, *Aphorisms*, 1883

Two minds are better than one

If you've been married for a long time, you may know instinctively what your partner is thinking. But did you know that your partner can help improve your thinking?

One study of couples who had been married more than 40 years found that, when allowed to work together, the older couples recalled as much information as younger couples or younger individuals. The people in the study listened to stories and then were asked to recall information about the stories both individually and as a couple.

Young people usually remember more correct story information than older people. However, when the older couples combined forces, they showed a much greater improvement over their individual recall than younger couples did.

The researcher in charge of the study, psychologist Roger Dixon, thinks that older people compensate for declines in individual memories by making more of social interactions.

Strangers who were assigned to work together also improved their recall ability, but not as much as married couples.

If you think you have a marriage made in heaven, hold onto it. It may help you hold onto your mental youthfulness.

7 ways to maintain mental muscle

One of the largest aging studies ever done, the Seattle Longitudinal Study, identified seven common factors among people who kept their mental sharpness as they aged.

- A willingness to change

- A high standard of living with an above average income and education

- Being married to an intelligent person

- A lack of chronic disease

- Satisfaction with accomplishments

- An ability to understand new ideas quickly

- Staying active — reading, traveling, continuing education, attending cultural events like theater, and participating in clubs and professional organizations

If you are fortunate enough, or smart enough, to possess all of the above qualities, congratulations. You should maintain that smart brain for years to come.

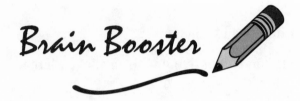

All hands on deck!

This puzzle will keep your brain in ship-shape. How many of these words ending in "ship" do you recognize? Example: You have to join the crew on this craft. If you answered "membership," you are ready to set sail. Bon voyage!

1. Not your best ship
2. Your aunts and uncles are aboard
3. A bright boy's boat
4. Not an easy ship to navigate
5. Your pal's vessel
6. You live and pay taxes here
7. Not a craft for aliens
8. Other ships follow
9. A carpenter's boat, perhaps
10. Traveling merchant ship
11. This one's a winner
12. You bought it

Check your answers in the *Solutions to Brain boosters and teasers* section at the back of the book.

Depression

Natural ways to beat the blues

Your brain is in control. It controls your thoughts, your movements, and even your moods and behavior. Sometimes, your brain doesn't do its job well, and the result is a mental disorder like depression.

If you have a disease of the body, it is usually easier to recognize, accept, and sometimes easier to treat than a disease of the mind. If you have a broken leg, no one would tell you to just "get over it." But if you suffer from depression, obsessive-compulsive disorder, or panic disorder, many people would say just that.

Obviously, there is more to it than just "pulling yourself up by your bootstraps." Depression and other mental illnesses have a physical basis, and a disorder of the mind can be just as painful as any broken bone. Just because no one else can see or feel it doesn't mean it isn't real.

"The diseases of the mind are more destructive than those of the body."
— Marcus Tullius Cicero

How to tell if it's depression

Your bank statement has a minus sign in front of the balance, every major appliance in your house is on the fritz, you had a fight with your best friend, your electric bill is past due, it's raining, and your dog just growled at you. It's enough to make a person depressed.

Into each life a little rain must fall, but sometimes it feels like you're in the middle of monsoon season. While it's normal for people to get a little "down" when life hands them the fuzzy end of the lollipop, real depression is an illness. Fortunately, it can be treated.

Sometimes events in your life make you feel blue. Some situational sadness is normal, but if you can't snap out of the depression, or if you feel depressed for no apparent reason, you may be in trouble. And you won't be alone. The National Institute of Mental Health (NIMH) estimates that more than 9 million Americans suffer from clinical depression.

To help you distinguish between just feeling blue and being clinically depressed, check out these symptoms of depression listed by the NIMH.

- Persistent sad, anxious, or "empty" mood

- Feelings of hopelessness, pessimism

- Feelings of guilt, worthlessness, helplessness

- Loss of interest or pleasure in hobbies and activities that were once enjoyed, including sex

- Insomnia, early-morning awakening, or oversleeping

- Appetite and/or weight loss or overeating and weight gain

- Decreased energy, fatigue, being "slowed down"

- Thoughts of death or suicide, suicide attempts

- Restlessness, irritability

- Difficulty concentrating, remembering, making decisions

- Persistent physical symptoms that do not respond to treatment, such as headaches, digestive disorder, and chronic pain

If these symptoms describe you, then you may be suffering from serious depression. See your doctor for a complete check-up to rule out physical problems, then seek professional help.

Fish oil — a fat that fights depression

Don't be offended if someone calls you a fathead. You're in good company. Albert Einstein, Thomas Edison, Sir Isaac Newton, and Confucius can be called fatheads, too. That's because fat makes up about 60 percent of the human brain.

But you do have a choice over what type of fathead you want to be. You can keep your brain running smoothly with the right kinds of fats or you can gum up the works with too much of the wrong kind. It all depends on what you eat.

Sound fishy? As a matter of fact, it is. The essential fats found in seafood, called omega-3 fatty acids, play a major role in brain function. They may even boost your mood.

Defeat depression. Next time you're feeling blue, dip into the deep blue sea for your dinner. New medical evidence suggests that the omega-3 fatty acids found in fish — called docosahexaenoic acid (DHA) and eicosapentaenoic acid (EPA) — can help drive away depression.

Dr. Andrew Stoll, a Harvard psychiatrist, found that fish oil capsules helped people with bipolar disorder, or manic depression. People with this condition go through periods of extreme highs and lows. During a high period, they might engage in reckless behavior like spending large sums of money foolishly, while during a low spell they might not get out of bed.

In his study, Dr. Stoll gave fish oil capsules to 14 people with bipolar disorder and a placebo to 16 others. Only 13 percent of the people taking the fish oil capsules experienced any return of depression or mania, compared with 52 percent for the placebo group. And the people taking the fish oil capsules performed significantly better than the placebo group on every test given to measure levels of depression.

According to Dr. Stoll, "The striking difference in relapse rates and response appeared to be highly clinically significant."

Dr. Stoll suggests that the omega-3 fatty acid in the fish oil capsules may act by slowing down neurons in the brain, similar to the drug Lithium, which is used to treat manic depression.

"Although the data are preliminary, our study indicates omega-3 fatty acids are safe and beneficial for patients with bipolar disorder," Dr. Stoll said. "Our finding opens the door for more research on omega-3 fatty acid's effect on a variety of other psychiatric disorders, including major depression, schizophrenia, and attention deficit hyperactivity disorder."

Plenty of other researchers have found links between omega-3 fatty acids and depression. One group from Sheffield, England, noticed that depressed people had much fewer omega-3 fatty acids in their red blood cells than healthy people. The more severe the depression, the less omega-3.

Dr. Joseph Hibbeln of the National Institutes of Health (NIH) in Bethesda, Md., reported similar findings in people across different cultures. For example, in Japan, where annual fish consumption is quite high (over 140 pounds per person), the rate of major depression is only .12 percent. That's a little more than one person with major depression out of every 1,000. On the other hand, in New Zealand, where people eat less than 40 pounds of fish per year, the rate of major depression is 5.8 percent, or 58 per 1,000.

Even though this doesn't prove that eating fish makes you less depressed, the evidence still packs a wallop.

"I am impressed that the two are so closely related," Dr. Hibbeln said. "I was very surprised at the power of the relationship, and I have been impressed that the relationship exists not only for major depression but also appears to exist for other depressive disorders."

There is even evidence that EPA can help treat people with schizophrenia, a serious mental illness that can cause delusions, hallucinations, and disorganized behavior.

Why does fish seem to fight depression? That's a good question without a definite answer. But science provides some strong ideas.

Neurotransmitters, the brain's Pony Express riders that carry messages from cell to cell, have an easier time wriggling through fat membranes made of fluid omega-3 than any other kind of fat. This means your brain's important messages get delivered, not denied access by membranes made of thick, hard fat.

Plus, eating fish has an effect on the levels of serotonin, one of your brain's good-news messengers. People with low levels of serotonin are more likely to be depressed, violent, and suicidal. If you have low levels of DHA, you also have low levels of serotonin. More DHA means more serotonin.

Most antidepressants, including Prozac, raise brain levels of serotonin. You might be doing the same thing just by eating fish. In other words, gills may be as good as pills.

Rethink your ratio. Whether you're depressed or not, chances are you should work more omega-3 into your diet. But it's not as simple as that. You'll probably also have to cut down on omega-6, another type of essential fatty acid found in vegetable oils, meat, milk, and eggs.

Omega-3 and omega-6 are polyunsaturated fatty acids your brain needs but can't make on its own.

"Essential fatty acids only appear through your diet," said Dr. William Lands of the NIH. "What you eat makes you what you are. You can't make 'em. So if you got 'em, it means you ate 'em."

Right now, the typical American eats at least 10 times more omega-6 than omega-3, or a ratio of 10-to-1. Some people's diets push that ratio to 25-to-1 or even higher.

It wasn't always that way. According to Dr. Hibbeln, thousands of years ago ancient people possibly ate five times more omega-3 than omega-6. And who ever heard of a depressed caveman?

But diets changed as people switched from hunting and gathering to an industrial society. They began eating less fruits, vegetables, and fish and more grain and farm-raised meat, not to mention processed foods. It's a menu that put the omega-6 to omega-3 ratio out of whack.

Not that omega-6 is bad. But when one type of fatty acid so outnumbers the other, things can go haywire. Too much omega-6 leads to too much signaling in your brain. With all the hyperactive omega-6 signals running wild, your brain becomes a house full of rowdy teenagers with the parents away for the weekend. This chaos can lead to headaches, arthritis, asthma, arrhythmia, and more. When you take aspirin or ibuprofen, you're getting rid of your headache by cutting down on the excessive omega-6 signaling.

Fortunately, the calmer omega-3 — the parents — can also stop the crazy antics of omega-6 and bring things back to normal. But omega-3 can only do so much in the face of such odds.

Go fish. So, you know why you need to fix your balance of omega-6 and omega-3. But how do you go about doing it?

The obvious first step is to eat more fish. Fatty fish like salmon, herring, mackerel, and tuna offer the most omega-3, but all seafood contains at least some. That's because all fish either eat marine algae, which is rich in the omega-3 fatty acids DHA and EPA, or gobble up other smaller fish that ate the algae.

Aim for at least two fatty fish meals per week. It will also protect your heart. In fact, the American Heart Association recommends two fish meals per week in its dietary guidelines. But if you have heart disease, the suggested number of fish meals per week jumps to seven.

If you're an absolute landlubber who can't stand fish, you can get some omega-3's by eating flaxseed; walnuts; and collard, turnip, and mustard greens. Other good sources include dark green, leafy vegetables like spinach, arugula, kale, Swiss chard, certain types of lettuce, and purslane, a hard-to-find green used in Mediterranean salads.

However, the omega-3 in these foods is in the form of alpha-linolenic acid, which the brain can convert to DHA only in small amounts. So, to get the good stuff your brain prefers, the pre-formed DHA and EPA, you still need to eat fish. Or you can take fish oil supplements, which are available in health food stores, pharmacies, and supermarkets. (Just one caution — if you're taking blood thinners, you might want to check with your doctor before taking supplements because omega-3 also has a blood-thinning effect.)

"I try to eat at least two to three meals of fish a week, and when I don't eat fish, I try to take supplements," Dr. Hibbeln said.

Just as important are the things he tries not to eat, namely soybean and corn oils, both much too high in omega-6 and too low in omega-3.

"You can do that a number of ways," Dr. Hibbeln said. "One is to completely eliminate all deep-fried foods from your diet. They're bad. Secondly, is to try to eliminate margarine and salad dressings that have corn or soybean oil in them."

Switching from corn or soybean oil to canola oil, which has a more favorable 2-to-1 ratio of omega-6 to omega-3, or to olive oil, a monounsaturated oil with the least amount of omega-6, would do wonders for your essential fatty acid balance.

(continued on page 264)

Grams of fatty acid per 100 grams (about 1/2 cup or 3 1/2 ounces) of food

Food	Omega-6 fatty acids	Omega-3 fatty acids ALA	EPA	DHA
Beans and legumes				
Lentils, dry	0.4	0.16	–	–
Lima beans, dry	0.5	0.2	–	–
Navy beans, dry	0.2	0.3	–	–
Pinto beans, cooked	0.2	0.3	–	–
Soybeans, cooked	0.4	2.1	–	–
Dairy and fats				
Butter	1.8	1.2	–	–
Cheese, cheddar	0.5	0.4	–	–
Cream, whipping	0.9	0.5	–	–
Egg, yolk	4.2	0.1	0	0
Margarine, hard, soybean	19.4	1.5	–	–
Mayonnaise, soybean	37.1	4.2	–	–
Milk, whole	–	0.1	–	–
Salad dressing, commercial, Italian	24.7	3.3	–	–
Fish and seafood				
Anchovy	0.2	–	0.5	0.9
Bluefish	0.4	–	0.4	0.8
Carp	0.8	0.3	.02	.01
Cod, Atlantic	Trace	Trace	0.1	.02
Crab, Alaska king	–	Trace	0.2	0.1
Flounder	0.1	Trace	0.1	0.1
Halibut, Pacific	0.2	0.1	0.1	0.3
Herring, Pacific	0.6	0.1	1.0	0.7
Mackerel, Atlantic	1.1	0.1	0.9	1.6
Salmon, Atlantic	0.7	0.2	0.3	0.9
Scallop, sea	0.6	0.3	21.3	26.2
Shrimp	0.2	Trace	O.2	0.1
Sole, lemon	0.7	2.0	14.7	6.8
Tuna, albacore	0.3	0.2	0.3	1.0
Fruit				
Avocados, California, raw	1.9	0.1	–	–
Raspberries	0.2	.01	–	–

Food	Omega-6 fatty acids	Omega-3 fatty acids		
		ALA	EPA	DHA
Grain				
Barley, bran	2.4	0.3	–	–
Oats, germ	11.0	1.4	–	–
Rice, bran	6.4	0.2	–	–
Wheat, bran	2.2	0.2	–	–
Wheat, germ	5.9	0.7	–	–
Meat and poultry				
Beef, ground, raw	0.8	0.2	–	–
Beef, T-bone steak, lean, raw	0.3	Trace	–	–
Chicken, light meat	0.4	Trace	Trace	0.02
Nuts and seeds				
Cashews	7.3	0.2	0	0
Flaxseed	7	17	0	0
Peanut	14.4	0.6	0	0
Walnuts, black	34.2	3.3	–	–
Oils				
Canola (rapeseed)	22.2	11.2	–	–
Cod liver	6.6	0.7	9.0	9.5
Flaxseed (linseed)	15	55	0	0
Olive	9	0.7	0	0
Peanut	29	1.1	0	0
Safflower	77	1	–	–
Soybean	53	7	0	0
Walnut	52.9	10.4	–	–
Wheat germ	54.8	6.9	–	–
Vegetables				
Broccoli, raw	0.03	0.1	–	–
Cauliflower, raw	–	0.1	–	–
Corn, germ	17.7	0.3	–	–
Kale, raw	0.1	0.2	–	–
Lettuce, Butterhead, raw	–	0.1	–	–
Mustard	–	0.04	–	–
Purslane	0.09	0.4	–	–
Seaweed, Spirulina, dried	1.2	0.8	–	–
Spinach, raw	0.1	0.9	–	–

"Just by throwing away that bottle and putting a new bottle in the kitchen, it makes a big difference."

The same advice — eat more fatty fish, substitute olive or canola oil for other vegetable oils, reduce deep-fried foods — appears in the book *The Omega Diet* by Dr. Artemis P. Simopoulos.

Her book includes recipes and tips for balancing your omega-6 to omega-3 ratio as well as sample three-week menus for breakfast, lunch, and dinner. What jumps out is just how much variety there is in a healthy, balanced diet.

That's also one of the points Dr. Lands has been trying to stress. "On a given day, you can really pig out on something," he said. "But with 30-some days in a month, you've got the rest of the month to atone for a given day's imbalance. Your body will integrate these things over time."

So know what you're eating, because it all boils down to this — what type of fat you eat determines how your brain works. Moreover, your food determines your mood. Just by getting more omega-3 and less omega-6 into your diet, you can put your brain, and your spirits, in high gear.

And that's no fish story.

A fishy solution for migraines

If you 've been fishing around for a solution to your migraines, maybe you should consider fish. Researchers at the University of Cincinnati gave fish oil capsules containing omega-3 fatty acids to migraine sufferers. About 60 percent of the people in the study reduced the frequency as well as the severity of their headaches.

Antidepressants — mood pills for the 90s

The mood ring was a popular fad in the 70s. Remember how you anxiously waited to see if the stone in your ring would change color and predict how you were feeling? Although no one really believed it worked, everyone still steered clear if your ring turned black, just in case.

Today "mood pills" might seem to be a fad. You can change your mood according to the pill you take. Unlike mood rings, however, most people have no doubt that mood pills work.

You have chemicals called neurotransmitters in your brain that help your brain cells communicate. Research finds that the brains of depressed people are a bit low on some of these chemicals. Serotonin, in particular, produces feelings of calmness and contentment. That is why most antidepressants work on increasing the serotonin levels in your brain.

The Prozac connection. You may have heard of the popular antidepressant, Prozac, a type of selective serotonin reuptake inhibitor (SSRI). Others include Paxil and Zoloft. These medications keep serotonin circulating in your brain so that your brain cells can use it longer. They are wonderful at relieving symptoms of depression, but they do have side effects. The most common are anxiety, insomnia, and weight loss. Others may include drowsiness, fatigue, tremor, sweating, upset stomach, decreased sex drive, and dizziness. You shouldn't take SSRIs with other antidepressants, especially MAO inhibitors.

Serotonin helpers. Monoamine oxidase (MAO) is a substance that eats up the extra serotonin in your brain. Obviously, that's not good. MAO inhibitors prevent it from doing that so more serotonin can get to your brain cells. The most serious side effect is severe high blood pressure. If you are taking one of these drugs, have your blood pressure checked often, and tell your doctor if you experience other side effects of high blood pressure. These include heart palpitations, frequent headaches, chest pain, enlarged pupils, and dizziness or lightheadedness when rising from a sitting or lying position. Most side effects, however, aren't severe and may go away with continued use. These include drowsiness, tremors, dry mouth, weight gain, fluid retention, and sexual disturbances.

Symptom fighters. Tricyclics are a group of antidepressants that help battle the symptoms of depression. They raise the amount of serotonin or norepinephrine, another neurotransmitter, in your central nervous system. But be careful. They can act like sedatives and make you drowsy, at least for the first few weeks. Other common side effects include dizziness, dry mouth, headache, increased appetite, nausea, and weight gain.

If your doctor prescribes antidepressants for you, be patient. It may take a few weeks before you can tell any difference in your mood. Never take more than one kind of antidepressant at a time, and be aware that they may stay in your system for a few weeks after you stop taking them. You also shouldn't drink alcohol when taking most antidepressants.

Natural miracle mood lifter

The millions of dollars spent on prescriptions for Prozac and Zoloft prove they are two of the most well-known and popular antidepressants in the United States. In a recent year, Americans spent almost $2.5 billion on these two drugs alone. Obviously, anyone suffering from major depression will gladly pay whatever it takes to feel better.

But although these and other antidepressants are effective, they can cost more than just money. Unwelcome side effects like insomnia, weight gain, and loss of sex drive may be almost as bad as the depression itself.

Luckily, you have an alternative that costs just pennies a day, doesn't require a prescription, and has few side effects. For many people, a plant called St. John's wort (*hypericum perforatum*) is a "miracle mood lifter" that provides the same relief from depression as prescription antidepressants.

Europeans have used the yellow flowering tops of St. John's wort for centuries. Hippocrates himself supposedly recommended it for a variety of ailments.

If you have mild to moderately severe depression, St. John's wort may help. Modern studies have found that extracts of hypericum effectively relieve those types of symptoms. It works like an MAO inhibitor, preventing the MAO enzyme from eating up your serotonin, thus making more of that "feel-good" chemical available to your brain.

The recommended daily dose is based on the amount of hypericin in the extract. If you take an extract that is standardized to contain 0.3 percent hypericin, the usual dosage would be 300 milligrams three times a day.

One warning: If you're looking forward to a summer tan, you'd better skip the sunbathing while taking this herb. St. John's wort may make your skin more sensitive to ultraviolet light. Try to stay out of strong sunlight, and also avoid tanning beds. And don't ever take it in combination with other antidepressant medications.

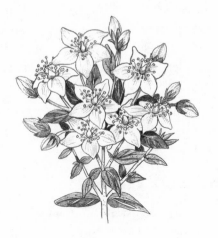

The simple yellow flowers of St. John's wort may provide inexpensive relief from depression.

Shake a leg to shake the blues

You know regular exercise will tighten and tone your body. If you doubt it, just look at the pictures on the covers of exercise videos. The instructor always has a smooth, slim body, which was sculpted by years of aerobics or sports. But did you know that exercise may also be responsible for her bubbly personality? Research finds exercise can improve your mind and your mood as well as your body.

One study tested a group of college professors before and after a six-week exercise program. There was no doubt that exercise helped lower depression levels. And, according to another study, aerobic exercise may be the best type to take up. Researchers found that 10 weeks of aerobic exercise lowered depression much more than just stretching. The extra oxygen that flows to your brain when you're running or swimming, for example, may help to lift your mood.

Regular exercise might also have a protective effect in people who are not depressed. One study of college students found that those who were fit were less likely to become depressed over the stresses of college life than those who got little exercise.

Run, walk, jump, or dance your way out of depression. It may be an effective, wholesome alternative to more expensive treatments. One study found that running improved depression levels as much as psychotherapy. Even though running shoes have gotten expensive, it's still much cheaper than psychotherapy, and you can benefit your body and your mind at the same time. So lace up those sneakers and shake a leg.

'Orange' you much calmer?

Do you love the smell of an orange just as you peel the skin back from the juicy sections? Japanese researchers have discovered that citrus fragrances may do more than make your mouth water. They may help ease depression.

Researchers found that rats who were exposed to citrus fragrances were calmer during stress tests. They also found that people being treated for depression could significantly reduce their doses of antidepressants if they applied citrus fragrance.

This was one small study, so don't throw away your antidepressants and plant an orange grove. However, a little lemon-scented air freshener couldn't hurt, and it might just calm your anxiety and perk you up.

Check your neck for a hidden cause of depression

If you have symptoms of depression, maybe you should check out your neck. According to the American Association of Endocrinologists, millions of Americans who think they're suffering from clinical depression may actually have thyroid disease.

Your thyroid is a small, butterfly-shaped gland in your neck that produces hormones that regulate your metabolism. It also has an important effect on organs like your brain, heart, liver, kidneys, and skin.

When your thyroid gland produces too much or not enough hormone, you may have symptoms similar to depression. However, over the last two years, only one in five people who have these types of symptoms have been tested for thyroid disease.

Hypothyroidism occurs when your thyroid doesn't produce enough thyroid-stimulating hormone (TSH). Your metabolism slows down; you feel sluggish and drained; and your skin may become dry, yellowish, and cold. Your voice may become hoarse, and you might start to lose your hair. This condition is easily treated with synthetic hormones.

When your thyroid is overactive, you have hyperthyroidism. You may feel anxious, "wired" but tired; your hands may tremble, and you may sweat more than usual. You may also have vision problems, heart palpitations, sleep disturbances, and more frequent bowel movements.

Hyperthyroidism can increase your risk of heart disease and osteoporosis. It can be treated by surgically removing part of your thyroid or by destroying part of it with radiation.

If you have the symptoms of depression, you can perform a simple self-examination of your thyroid. Just look in a mirror, tip your head back, and drink a glass of water. As you swallow, look for signs of an enlarged or irregular thyroid gland. It is located just above your collarbone below your Adam's apple. Your doctor also can perform a test that will determine the level of TSH in your blood.

Left untreated, thyroid disease can cause serious, long-lasting problems. More than half of the estimated 13 million people in the United States who have the disease don't know it. Don't be one of the uninformed. Find out if you have the disorder, have it treated, and your depression may slip away forever.

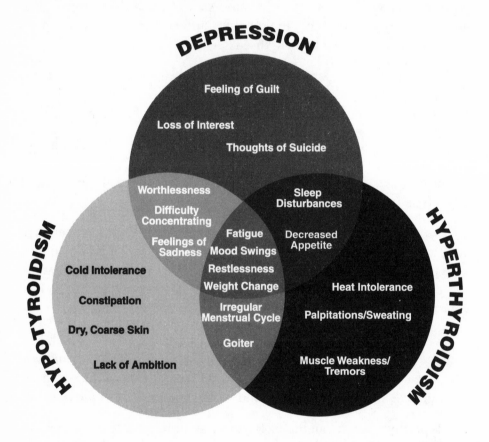

An easy way to rub out depression

A massage can bring relief from tense, tired, sore muscles. It may also bring relief from depression.

A study supported by the National Institute of Mental Health found that massage therapy eased depression and anxiety and reduced levels of stress hormones like cortisol. Massage also stimulates your brain to produce more endorphins, chemicals that help block pain and increase your sense of well-being.

A soothing massage can invigorate you, physically and mentally, so check out your local massage therapist, and rub out depression for good.

Stop the heart-breaking cycle

Depression can be a heart-breaking illness, literally. It can raise your risk of heart disease.

Doctors have known that depression can slow a person's recovery from a heart attack. But surprising new research finds that it may also contribute to heart disease. In one study, people who scored high on a depression test had a 70 percent higher risk of heart attack. They also had a 60 percent higher risk of death compared to people who had low symptoms of depression.

Another heart disease link is high blood pressure. Depression and anxiety may raise your blood pressure, which also could lead to heart problems.

Of course, the reverse may be true as well. You might be depressed because you have heart disease, especially if you're older. The two diseases may feed off one another, creating an endless cycle.

Luckily, you can control both these illnesses. Lifestyle changes like eating right, exercising, and reducing stress can help protect you from the heartbreak of depression and the sadness of heart disease.

Special goggles make the world rosier

Optimistic people may be accused of viewing the world through rose-colored glasses, but one study finds that how you view the world may indeed affect your mood.

Researchers gave people in psychotherapy special goggles that allowed them to see only out of the far left or far right side of their visual field. Other people were given goggles that didn't affect their vision.

More than half of the people with depression reported more anxiety when looking out of the left side of their vision, which is controlled by the right side of the brain. However, a surprising number of those with post-traumatic stress syndrome were more anxious when looking out of the right side. This was unusual since the left brain (which controls the right side) is usually considered less emotional.

In any case, the study found that people who wear the goggles consistently tend to see the world in a more positive light when looking out of only one side.

Researchers aren't sure what these results mean yet, but they'll be doing more studies on the goggles, and someday mood-lifting glasses may be the hottest thing since Ben Franklin's bifocals.

Breakthrough treatment battles severe depression

Magnets attract metals, but they also may provide a more attractive way to treat severe depression than the long-time practice of electric shock therapy.

You've probably seen movies where mentally ill patients are treated with electric shocks. It's a disturbing image, even though the use of electricity to treat medical problems goes back to ancient times. The Roman Emperor Claudius was treated for headaches by pressing electric eels to his temples. Still, the idea of electroconvulsive therapy (ECT), or shock therapy, may be shocking to some people.

Nevertheless, ECT may be the answer for people with severe depression who don't respond to medication. It has probably saved many from suicide. But the treatment does sometimes cause serious side effects, including memory loss. Magnets may provide the same benefits without the complications involved in ECT.

How does the new technology work? An electromagnetic coil sends magnetic pulses into the brain. Unlike electricity, which spreads throughout the skull, the pulses can be directed at specific areas such as the left prefrontal cortex. This is a site of unusually low metabolism in depressed people, and the magnetic stimulation seems to speed it up. The procedure can be done while the person is awake, whereas ECT needs to be done under anesthesia. The only reported side effect so far is a mild headache.

The use of magnetic stimulation is still in the experimental stages. But it shows promise as an alternative for depressed people who haven't been helped by other treatments.

> *"If you are physically sick,*
> *you can elicit the interest of a battery of physicians;*
> *but if you are mentally sick,*
> *you are lucky if the janitor comes around."*
> — Martin H. Fischer

Women: save your bones from depression

Women may have more to fear from depression than men. According to statistics, major depression affects about twice as many women as men.

Depression may also increase the risk of another disease women fear — osteoporosis. Women get this bone-breaking disease much more often than men. It causes your bones to become less dense and weaker until the slightest impact can shatter them.

A study by the National Institute of Mental Health found that women with depression had bone density that was 10 to 15 percent lower than other women their age. They think it's probably because they have too much cortisol, a hormone the brain sends out in response to stress. Researchers already know you have a higher risk of osteoporosis if you use corticosteroids, a medicine similar to cortisol, for a long time.

Fighting depression can make you stronger emotionally. It may also make your bones stronger, capable of carrying you through years of happiness.

Brighten up a SAD syndrome

When you were a kid, you probably hated to see the sun go down. It meant you had to stop playing and go inside. If you're one of the millions of adults with seasonal affective disorder (SAD), you may now have even more reason to dread sundown.

Seasonal affective disorder affects 10 to 25 million people in the United States. It tends to set in during the winter when daylight hours become shorter. If you live in the north, you're even more likely to get it. Find yourself sluggish, depressed, and constantly craving sweets? Check the calendar — you may have SAD.

Researchers think SAD occurs in some people because the shortage of light throws off their circadian rhythms. If you think you may be affected by SAD, follow these tips and brighten up your life.

Wake up to the light. Change your sleep pattern so you are awake in the morning and exposed to as much early daylight as possible. Morning sunshine increases the level of melatonin in your body, a hormone that helps regulate your sleep cycle naturally. So open your blinds or curtains and let the sunshine help you get out of bed and into a better mood.

Take a walk. Make a point of getting outside every day. A daily walk will expose you to sunlight, and the exercise may give you a boost, too.

Raise the shades. The weather or your health may force you to remain indoors a lot during the winter, but you can still let some light in. Open the drapes, raise the shades, and turn on lights in windowless rooms.

Try some light in a box. Your doctor may prescribe light therapy for a severe case of SAD. This usually consists of a metal box with fluorescent lights inside. You set it on a desk or table and sit in front of it for 30 minutes to an hour every day. This is supposed to reset your circadian rhythm through light entering your eyes. However, a recent study found that light shining on the back of the knees was also effective in resetting circadian rhythms. Researchers are now conducting more experiments to determine if shining light on the backs of your knees while you are asleep can help with SAD.

Don't stock up on sweets. Most people with SAD eat more during the winter, particularly sweets. This often results in weight gain, which can be depressing itself. If you know you are susceptible to this, don't keep sweets on hand, so you won't be tempted to indulge whenever you're feeling "down."

Put the squeeze on stress. Stress can make the symptoms of SAD worse, so try to keep stress under control. See the *Mindpower* chapter for more information on stress management.

If you have SAD, there's no reason to just accept being depressed for half the year. Any steps you take to control SAD are steps toward a happier winter and a happier life.

*"The greatest barrier to love is the secret fear that we are unlovable.
The greatest barrier to happiness is the wordless sense
that happiness is not our proper destiny."*

— Nathaniel Branden

Help yourself to a healthier mind

If you have a sprained ankle or the flu, you probably know exactly where to go for professional medical help. If you have a mental problem like depression, however, your choice may not be so clear.

Most people who have emotional or mental problems never seek professional help. Maybe they don't know where to go, or perhaps they don't believe therapy helps.

However, according to a survey by Consumer Reports, therapy does help most people. The people surveyed reported being satisfied with help from social workers, psychologists, psychiatrists, family doctors, and self-help groups like Alcoholics Anonymous.

Even though you know therapy will probably help, you may still be confused about what kind of therapist is best for you. Here's a quick overview of the most common types of therapists.

- **Psychiatrists** — Medical doctors who have been trained to diagnose any illness, but have special training in treating emotional problems. They can prescribe medicine for any disorder.

- **Psychologists** — They have doctoral-level training in psychology, not medicine. They cannot prescribe medicine, but in some situations, they may recommend a medication and refer you to a medical doctor.

- **Psychoanalysts** — Specialize in analyzing the unconscious mind. Their approach to treatment is that mental problems are caused by life experiences.

- **Social workers** — Usually trained in a wide range of social services. They may be state licensed or certified.

- **Marriage and family therapists** — May have a professional degree with supervised experience in their specialty.

If you've decided that therapy may be just what you need, you can ask your doctor for a referral, or ask your family and friends for recommendations. You can also call your county mental health department or your local or state psychological association.

Don't be afraid to check credentials and ask questions when choosing a therapist. Ask if they are licensed and how many years they've been practicing. Find out if they have experience with your type of problem, and what kind of treatments they prefer for your problem. Prices can vary greatly among different types of therapists, and so can insurance coverage, so be sure to ask about those issues, too.

Don't think that your first choice has to be your last, either. You probably wouldn't dream of buying the first car you looked at unless it was the perfect car for you, and the choice of a therapist is so much more important. Sometimes you just don't "click" with a particular therapist, so shop around until you find one you trust. By making an appropriate choice, you'll go a long way toward helping yourself recover.

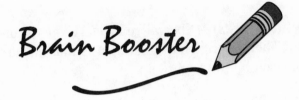

Mental mix-up

Boost your brain power and your mood by keeping your brain occupied. Unscramble these words from this chapter.

esridpsnoe _____   odom _____

zcrapo _____   sgemasa _____

cxeesrei _____   setsrs _____

ionasmin _____   xeitnay _____

erhat esadies _____   eatihpstr _____

trohpmyhidsiyo _____   ts hjosn rowt _____

odlob srespuer _____

stiumrnosertrtane _____

naselaso eftavfcie sedorrid _____

Check your answers in the *Solutions to Brain boosters and teasers* section at the back of the book.

Headache

Heading off the misery

Headsplitter. Jackhammer. Brain pain.

There are lots of different names for a headache, but they all mean the same thing — your head is pounding so hard you can't see straight. A headache can bring you a few minutes of annoyance or can knock you out for days at a time.

Is it actually your brain that hurts, or does a headache just happen to be in that area? Frankly, science hasn't completely answered that question yet, but researchers learn more every year.

One theory is that headaches are caused by a chemical imbalance in your brain. Serotonin, a brain chemical involved in transmitting pain messages in your brain, may be at the root of some headaches. Many headache medications work by regulating the action of serotonin.

One of the newer theories on migraines is that some people have brain cells that are abnormally excitable. When these overactive neurons are set off by a trigger, such as bright lights or irregular sleep patterns, they send out ripples of electrical energy. This, in turn, causes blood flow to surge and drop suddenly, resulting in pain.

However it happens, most experts agree that enlarged blood vessels pressing on brain tissue cause the pain in most headaches. For this reason, headache remedies seek to find those blood vessels and shrink them back down to size, taking the pressure and the pain away.

If you want to cure your headache naturally, that's what you must do, too. Headaches come in all shapes and sizes so figuring out which kind you have is the first step toward getting rid of it.

> *"When the head aches,*
> *all the body is the worse."*
>
> — English proverb

Don't let tension turn to pain

You were two hours late for work today because your car got a flat tire. Your boss yelled at you for someone else's mistake, and after work, you shopped for groceries for an hour before realizing you had forgotten your checkbook. At home, the toilet is overflowing, your taxes are due in three days, and the neighbor's dog won't stop barking.

What's throbbing through your head right now is called a tension headache. It's probably the most common kind to get because it's mostly caused by stress, something we all have plenty of. A tension headache usually attacks your whole head, making it feel sore and pressurized. The feeling is sometimes described as wearing a tight band all the way around your head.

Tension headaches don't usually last as long as other types, but the pain can be extreme. And depending on how you handle stress, they can come back quite often.

Self-help solutions. The best way to keep clear of tension headaches is to avoid tension. This is true for both prevention and treatment.

- De-stress your life as much as you can. Avoid things that cause you extreme stress or tend to upset you. If you feel yourself stressing out, practice relaxation techniques.

- Get regular exercise; it's a great stress-buster and good for you in many other ways, too.

- "Cool out" a tension headache with massage. Sit still with your eyes closed and rub your sore head. Work your fingers over your temples and forehead or wherever you feel pain. Rub your shoulders and neck to release the tightness that stress inflicts on your body. Breathe slowly and deeply, and concentrate on relaxing while you massage.

- Get relief from aspirin or ibuprofen. A recent study shows that combining aspirin with caffeine may do an even better job of stopping a tension headache.

- Apply heating or cooling pads to your head, whichever is more comfortable.

- Take a nap. Sometimes sleep is the only thing that will interrupt the pain cycle.

If you suffer frequently, the best idea is to experiment with several different methods until you find one form of relief that works consistently for you.

How to avert migraine agony

You walk out into a sunny day and suddenly your vision goes fuzzy. A zig-zaggy pattern of lights and stars crosses your eyes, and it feels like the world has a strange halo around it. A short time later, pain builds up in your head until the slightest move sends a throbbing pulse of agony shooting through your brain. Diagnosis: migraine.

This type of headache is one of the most painful you can experience. It usually comes as a throbbing, severe ache in the front or sides of your head and can last up to two or three days. In some cases, the pain can be bad enough to cause nausea, vomiting, and even diarrhea.

Sufferers of "classic" migraines know when they are about to get one because a halo, or "aura," appears to them. They may see patterns in the air or strange, glowing variations of light. People who suffer from migraines can get them on a regular basis or just once or twice a year. Like everything else about migraines, the frequency depends on each individual person.

Self-help solutions. No one knows for sure what causes migraines, but everyone agrees that certain things can trigger the painful attacks.

- A good way to fend off migraines, or at least to make them more bearable, is to keep track of your "triggers." Caffeine, alcohol, salty foods; just about anything can be a trigger, and knowing what brings your headaches on can help you avoid them. (See the *Dear diary* story.)

- When you get a migraine, stay out of the sun, and try to get some sleep. Migraine sufferers report that this is often the only thing that works.

- You can try hot towels or cold compresses, pressed to your head, or anything that makes you feel more comfortable.

- If your migraine has caused other symptoms, treat those as well. Drink lots of fluids if you have diarrhea, or settle a nauseous stomach with some ginger tea or flat cola.

Most migraine sufferers get these headaches more than once, so it's important to pinpoint what causes them. Find the method of relief that works for you, and stick with it. If it doesn't do the trick, then don't be afraid to talk to your doctor about other treatments.

Dear diary: Shaking free of migraine pain

To prevent migraines, you have to figure out what causes your migraine attacks. One of the best ways to do this is to keep a diary of possible triggers.

If you feel a migraine coming on, write down the foods you have recently eaten and the activities you are doing. Keep your diary up to date, writing down how bad each headache is and how long it lasts.

By comparing the information of several different headaches, you may be able to root out one or more of your triggers. For instance, if your diary shows that when you got your last three migraines you were either reading a book, walking your dog, or taking a nap, there's probably no pattern there.

However, if your diary's food column for your last three attacks reads chocolate cake, candy bar, and double-mocha ice cream, you may have discovered a very common trigger among migraine sufferers — chocolate.

And, unfortunately, you may just have to sacrifice this sweet treat to gain a migraine-free life.

'Cluster' buster strategies

It's 2 a.m. and you just woke up with a severe ache on one side of your head. The pain is burning, terrible, and it makes you dizzy as you stumble to the bathroom to look for some aspirin. The aspirin doesn't help, but after about an hour, the pain goes away and you go back to sleep, only to be awakened again 10 minutes later by another sharp, burning pain on that same side of your head.

Welcome to the excruciating world of cluster headaches. These headaches get their name from the fact that they come in bunches, or "clusters." If you get one, you're likely to suffer a few more, perhaps stretched out over a couple of days. The pain of a cluster headache is sharp, stabbing, and severe, and most people think it is even more painful than a migraine. The pain usually comes on one side of your head, but it can spread to affect your whole head, eyes, face, neck, or sometimes your whole upper body at once.

Cluster headaches don't last long, but they come back. Some sufferers can go for months, even years, without an attack, but when the clusters do return, it may be for as long as two weeks of on-again, off-again torture.

Self-help solutions. Although no one knows exactly what causes them, cluster headaches strike about six times more men than women, so it may have something to do with typical living styles.

- Many sufferers are heavy smokers and drinkers, so this gives you another reason to cut those habits out of your life.

- Since clusters strike mostly at night, getting on a regular sleep cycle can help.

- Putting an icepack or cold compress against your head can lessen the pain. As with other headaches, a heating pad may work better for you — experiment to find out.

- Some sufferers have success with the odd remedy of holding their hands in icewater until the hands become uncomfortable.

However you deal with your cluster, it's probably a good idea to see your doctor. Cluster headaches can be a symptom of a greater problem. Also, your doctor might be able to give you a prescription remedy that can handle your powerful headache.

Hidden causes of headache pain

Apart from the three main types of headaches — tension, migraine, and cluster — you may suffer a hundred different variations caused by a hundred different things. A head cold or allergies can fill your sinuses and cause a headache. Or if you skip a meal, hunger can put the pain in your brain. Heat, drugs, exhaustion, high blood pressure, and alcohol are also common causes.

Grinding your teeth while you sleep is another sneaky cause of daytime headaches. If you suspect this might be the source of your pain, have your dentist check your pearly whites for signs of grinding. Avoid chewing gum for a while to give your jaw a necessary rest, too.

Older adults have some special concerns in regard to their aching heads. As with others, a particularly bad or unusual headache can be a sign of a greater problem for an elderly person. Giant cell arthritis, for example, is a serious but largely treatable disorder, for which headache is a leading sign. If your other symptoms include muscle pain in the shoulders and hips, jaw pain when chewing, sweating, appetite and weight loss, and fever, you should have a blood test to check for this condition.

Hypnic headache is another uncommon but troublesome problem. A hypnic is a lot like a cluster headache, although generally not as painful. It wakes you up at night and doesn't last long but comes back after about a half hour.

Acute glaucoma, certain types of arthritis, and other ailments can cause headaches, primarily tension headaches. If you're taking medications to treat other conditions, they may trigger or worsen your headaches. By dealing with the pain from these other sources, you may be able to knock off that headache before it begins.

Surprising source of unexplained headaches

You've turned over a new leaf. You're going to really start looking out for your health. You're making some changes, and your first step is to cut out junk food and bad habits.

Then why, all of a sudden, are you getting those bad headaches every morning? Healthy is supposed to feel good, right?

Right, but maybe not all at once.

Was caffeine one of the "junk foods" you cut from your diet? If so, that may be your problem right there.

Caffeine withdrawal is a common cause of unexplained headaches. To prevent this unpleasantness, try to wean yourself off the magic bean instead of going cold turkey.

- Drink your coffee at the same time every day.

- Each day, drink a little less than the day before.

- Take your time.

If you take it slow, your brain has a chance to get used to less and less caffeine. And that means it will be less likely to take it out on you.

Fight back with ancient herbal remedy

Aspirin has been a traditional headache remedy for years and years. Pretty impressive, but has it been around for 20 centuries?

Two thousand years ago, ancient cultures like the Greeks had never heard of aspirin, but they had something better. It was a small herb called feverfew, and many people still use it today for many purposes, including putting their headaches out of commission.

Feverfew works to reduce inflammation and muscle spasms by keeping your body from releasing inflammatory chemicals. When you have a migraine, your brain releases the chemical serotonin, which can cause the blood vessels in your head to grow wider and irritate the nerve endings there. Feverfew helps prevent this from happening.

Feverfew has done well in clinical trials. In some tests, it has brought down the number and severity of migraines and also helped lessen vomiting. Unfortunately, it doesn't seem to affect how long they last.

If feverfew works for you, it can keep you out of the drugstore and probably save you some money. Most health food stores sell feverfew. Chewing two fresh leaves a day should be enough to chase off your headaches. A more convenient dose is in capsule form, but make sure it contains at least 0.2 percent parthenolide. That's the minimum standard for effectiveness.

Halt headaches with magnesium?

Are magnesium supplements the key to releasing you from your headache woes? That question is still up in the air.

Maybe you've heard about the research that suggests low levels of magnesium cause migraines. This news is partially true. Studies at the New York Headache Center have shown that as many as 50 percent of migraine and cluster headache sufferers have low levels of ionized magnesium. In several trials, people were given intravenous doses of extra magnesium, and many experienced relief from their headache pain.

But the doctors who ran these tests warn that this success does not mean headache sufferers should run out and start taking magnesium supplements.

First of all, there are many different kinds of magnesium on the market, and some can cause side effects such as diarrhea. Also, taking it every day can be expensive, and there is still no guarantee that extra magnesium will work. Finally, the doctors argue that putting too much hope in this method can keep you from trying to find a more effective solution to your headache problem.

So stay off the magnesium tablets. The best thing to do is try to eat a balanced diet and get your daily allowance of magnesium naturally.

Use your mind to soothe your pain

When a bad headache strikes, you probably wish you could just lie down, zone out, and forget the pain. Well, such a cure might be within your reach if you're willing to try something a little different. How about hypnosis?

The idea of hypnosis might scare you away because of its reputation for making people do silly things. But real hypnosis is simply the ability to relax your body and open your mind to the power of suggestion.

This ability has powerful healing uses because you can use it to suggest — and achieve — relief from muscle tension, stress, and headache pain.

Anyone can be hypnotized, but how effective the procedure is on you depends largely on how "open" you are to the idea of hypnotism. In other words, if you don't believe it will work, it almost certainly will not.

Some tips for relieving pain through hypnosis:

- Sit in a comfortable position and close your eyes. If you have a tension headache, think about the parts of your body, one by one, that feel tense. You may flex these stressed-out muscles, again one by one, and release. Breathe easily, and think about all the stress and tension dissolving in your muscles and leaving your body.

- Next, move your thoughts to your head. Focus on cool thoughts, soothing images that will ease your tight head. Use anything that helps to take away your stress, relax you, and make the pressure in your head go down.

Researchers say these techniques work best for people who know exactly what is causing their headache and can concentrate specifically on how the healing should happen. That means you should focus on the swollen blood vessels in your head that are causing the headache. Think of a great coolness in your head that is soothing those blood vessels. Picture these blood vessels shrinking — getting smaller, less pressurized, less painful.

Some people — even some doctors — are suspicious of hypnosis. But this is simply because these techniques are not traditional standard practice. So why not give your pocketbook a rest and the power of your mind a chance? If you're interested, you can find more on this type of therapy in the *Mindpower* chapter. By mastering the art of healing hypnosis, headache relief will never be more than a few quiet moments away.

'Baby' migraines away

Looking for a quick bite without any chemical additives or flavorings? Next time you're at the supermarket, head down an aisle you haven't visited in a while.

Some migraine sufferers swear that baby food is an efficient way to grab a quick meal while avoiding many of the food additives that can trigger attacks. If your doctor has recommended a restricted diet for you, it can be rather inconvenient to prepare "safe" meals all the time. A small jar of stewed prunes can be a reasonably tasty and nutritious way to tide you over until you can put together something a bit more substantial.

But don't take it too far. Some migraine sufferers who believe food additives are their only triggers stick to a strictly Gerber diet. One Chicago doctor notes that if a person's life is so busy he only has time for baby food, perhaps food additives aren't the only things causing his headaches. It might be a good idea to look at other ways to manage migraine pain as well.

Besides, strained carrots for supper? What would your dinner guests say?

7 warning signs of a serious problem

Headaches are inconvenient and can be extremely painful, but they are not usually dangerous. Sometimes, however, a headache can be a sign of a more serious problem. It's difficult to tell, but the best advice is to watch for anything different from what your headaches usually feel like. For example:

- Abrupt, very painful headache that hits hard.

- Headache accompanied by other symptoms, like fever, confusion, nausea, blurry vision.

- Head pain that causes you to pass out.

- Headache that doesn't go away after an infection or sore throat.

- Any headache that keeps up after an injury.

- A new type of headache pain after the age of 55.

- Anything different or worse than usual.

See your doctor as soon as a headache seems out of the ordinary. An unusual, persistent headache could be a symptom of a larger problem. Some of these, such as blood clots and tumors, are highly treatable but can be deadly if left alone for too long.

So when in doubt, check it out. It's better to play it safe than to risk missing a serious condition.

Relief runs hot and cold

Cold compresses and heating pads are two highly recommended ways to soothe a headache. But how can that be since they are opposites?

The truth is, everyone's headache is unique, so everyone will react differently to different treatments. Cold is probably used more often since the chill helps shrink swollen blood vessels that often cause pain. Regardless, chances are good that your headache pain will respond to either cold or warmth but probably not both. Simply figure out which works for you, and go with it.

Another bit of good news — these methods should give you some relief no matter what type of head pain you suffer from. So whether you respond to "fire" or "ice," you'll be on your way to a quicker recovery.

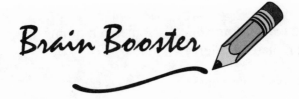

It's all in your head

Can you guess the word or phrase represented by each of the following drawings? They all contain the word "head."

1.

2.

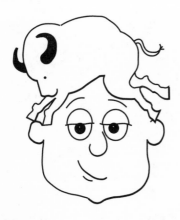

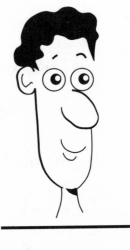

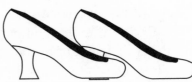

3.

4.

5.

6.

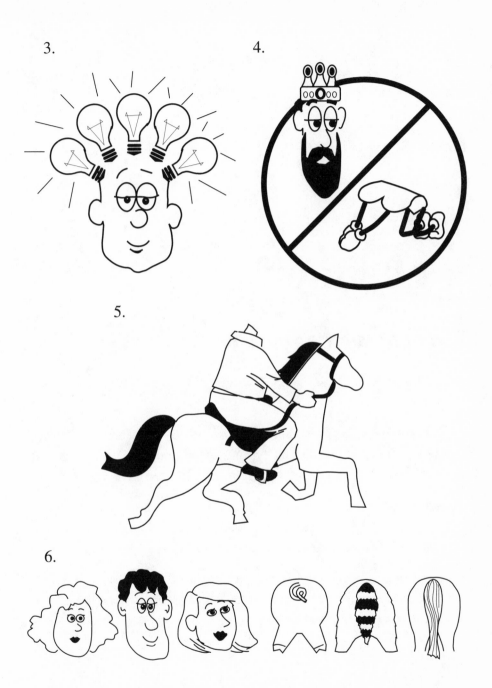

Check your answers in the *Solutions to Brain boosters and teasers* section at the back of the book.

Alzheimer's

How to hold onto your memories

Joan Hoffman looks at her husband of 45 years and has no idea who he is. She refers to him as "young man" and asks him to slow the car down, even though she's sitting in a recliner in their living room.

Alzheimer's disease is slowly stealing Joan's memories. Although she has moments and sometimes even hours of clear thoughts, most of the time she doesn't recognize her friends, family, or even her surroundings.

Alzheimer's can affect anyone, from an ordinary person like Joan, to a former President of the United States, Ronald Reagan. It may someday affect you or someone you love, so you need to learn all you can to help stop this disease in its tracks.

Diary of a dreaded disease

Look at your photo album, filled with reminders of days past — pictures of children, relatives, pets, vacations, and holidays. Now think how you would feel if you looked at those photos and had no memories of those occasions — if you didn't recognize the faces and places of your past.

If you're like most people, you fear Alzheimer's disease (AD) because it takes away your most precious possession — your mind. The fact that Alzheimer's is fatal almost doesn't matter.

Alzheimer's disease robs you of everything you've learned throughout your entire life, both mentally and physically. Over seven to 10 years, it gradually steals all your brain processes, including memory, language, judgment, behavior, personality, abstract thinking, and motor skills. You once again become as helpless as a baby. No wonder people find it frightening.

When pathologist Alois Alzheimer first discovered this disease in 1907, there was little hope for those suffering from it. Researchers couldn't even begin to unravel the mystery of the plaques and tangles found in unhealthy AD brain cells. But since then, science has plunged into the mysterious and complex world of the brain and discovered more than we ever thought possible about how our minds work.

So take heart. With the research and technology we have today, the possibility of treating, and even preventing, this mind-robbing disease may be just around the corner.

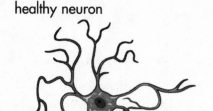

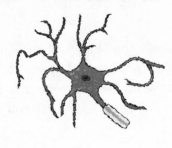

In Alzheimer's disease, brain cells lose many of their connections and processes.

Warning: 10 early signs of Alzheimer's

You tend to become more forgetful as you get older or busier. Every time you forget a name or lose your glasses, you may panic, thinking you have Alzheimer's. Chances are, you're perfectly fine. In fact, worrying about your memory loss is actually a good sign that you're OK. People with severe memory problems are usually unaware of their own lapses, so it may be up to family members to notice.

Unfortunately, a recent study found that one out of five families with a member who has mental problems were unable to recognize the problem. Detecting Alzheimer's early may help slow its progress, so look at this list of early warning signs that you or a loved one may have the disease.

Forgetfulness. The most well-known signal that you might have Alzheimer's is simply forgetfulness. While it's normal to forget names or lose your keys once in a while, frequent forgetfulness may be a red flag. The classic example is that it's normal to forget your keys, but if you can't remember what the keys are for, it's time to worry.

Speech problems. Sometimes a word is on the tip of your tongue, but you just can't get it out. Everyone has that experience occasionally, but if you often have trouble with simple words, or your speech isn't understandable, you may have a problem.

Misplacing things. Some people lose track of their keys or the TV remote control almost every day. But finding lost items in a strange place, like the microwave or the refrigerator, should be cause for concern.

Personality changes. Everyone goes through changes in their lives. Some people become more laid-back and relaxed as they age, while others seem to turn into grumpy old men and women. Alzheimer's can cause profound personality changes, making a calm, sweet person frightened, paranoid, or confused.

Loss of judgment. You may think young people show poor judgment in their choice of clothes, but if you can't judge what clothing is appropriate for you to wear, you may be the one with a problem. For example, if you put your socks on your hands, or wear shorts when it's snowing, you have lost your ability to judge.

Loss of interest. Everyone can lose interest in a slow-paced movie, but when you aren't interested in all the things that used to bring you pleasure, like hobbies, that's a little more serious.

Problems with familiar tasks. Busy people often are distracted and may forget to finish something they started. Someone with Alzheimer's might prepare a meal and not only forget to serve it, but not remember she even made it in the first place. Or she may have problems remembering how to prepare the meal at all.

Mood swings. Although many people are moody sometimes, going from one extreme to the other rapidly for no apparent reason is cause for concern.

Disorientation. If you get lost in a strange city, no one would accuse you of having Alzheimer's. If you get lost in your own neighborhood, that's another story. Place or time disorientation is an early symptom of Alzheimer's. If you easily forget what day it is or how to get to a familiar place, you should see a doctor.

Trouble "adding it up." Maybe math was your worst subject in school. Still, if doing simple math problems suddenly becomes more difficult, you may have a problem yourself. Math requires abstract thinking, connecting symbols (numbers) with a meaning. Abstract thinking is one of the first skills you lose with Alzheimer's.

Risky business: Who gets Alzheimer's?

Alzheimer's currently affects around 2 million people in the United States, with that figure expected to rise to almost 3 million by the year 2015. What are your chances of developing this disease? The risk factors involved can give you an idea.

Age. This is by far the biggest risk factor for Alzheimer's. Most people who get the disease are over 65, but don't let that spoil your hopes for a long, healthy life. Everyone who lives past 65 won't get AD. Only 5 to 6 percent of older people have it. With more people living longer, however, that means more and more people will be affected if scientists don't find a cure.

Family history. One study of Finnish twins found that if one identical twin developed Alzheimer's the other twin's chance of getting it was unusually high — about 40 to 50 percent. Another large study found that having two parents with Alzheimer's increased your risk to 54 percent by age 80, a five times greater risk than people whose parents did not have the condition.

Down syndrome. People born with this form of mental retardation almost always get Alzheimer's if they live long enough. Having a close relative with Down syndrome may also increase your risk.

Female sex. Alzheimer's affects more women than men at any age.

Head injury. A serious head injury may make you more likely to get Alzheimer's later in life.

These are the most well-established risk factors for Alzheimer's, but don't worry if you fall into some of these categories. You can't control your age, family history, or sex, but there are other things you can control that may help you avoid this disease.

healthy brain

brain with Alzheimer's disease

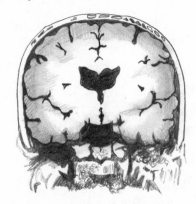 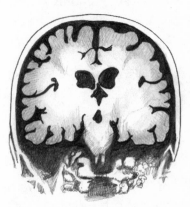

A brain with Alzheimer's has more space between the folds of the brain, an indication of lost brain tissue.

Over-the-counter prevention

Would you believe science has connected Alzheimer's with arthritis and leprosy? Fortunately, it's a good connection. Years ago, researchers noticed that people with arthritis rarely got Alzheimer's. And now, Japanese researchers also have discovered the same tendency among leprosy victims.

What's the link? Arthritis and leprosy are both treated with large daily doses of nonsteroidal anti-inflammatory drugs (NSAIDs). So researchers wondered if the treatment these people got for their conditions helped them avoid Alzheimer's.

No one knows for sure what causes Alzheimer's. Some experts think inflamed brain tissue might contribute to the plaques and tangles that are a sure sign of the disease. That means NSAIDs, which reduce swelling, may help prevent or treat the condition.

Several large studies have supported this theory. One study found that people who took ibuprofen (Advil and Motrin) more than occasionally were up to 60 percent less likely to get AD.

Johns Hopkins researchers studied people who already had Alzheimer's. They found that those who took NSAIDs, like ibuprofen and aspirin, progressed more slowly with the disease. They kept more of their cognitive skills, so they were able to function independently for a longer time.

A prescription drug for arthritis also could be a saving grace for Alzheimer's sufferers. Indomethacin has been found to help prevent or treat Alzheimer's. One exciting study found that it might even reverse some of the damage already caused by the disease. After six months, AD sufferers who took this drug showed a 1.3 percent improvement on cognitive tests, while people who didn't get the medicine had an 8.4 percent decline in mental function.

These promising and inexpensive remedies may be just what you need to stem the tide of Alzheimer's disease. However, NSAIDs can cause serious side effects, like stomach irritation and bleeding. Talk with your doctor before starting any treatment.

One-a-day way to put the brakes on Alzheimer's

A vitamin found in any drugstore may help you buy some time before Alzheimer's steals your health. This miracle vitamin, which a recent study found can slow the progression of AD, is the highly touted antioxidant, vitamin E.

Researchers divided people with Alzheimer's into four groups. They gave one group 2,000 international units (IU) of vitamin E daily. Another group took selegiline, a drug used to treat Parkinson's disease. The other groups got either a combination of vitamin E and selegiline or a placebo.

The people who took either the vitamin E or the selegiline were able to care for themselves longer and delayed entering a nursing home by about seven months, compared with the people who got the placebo.

The 2,000-IU dose of vitamin E used in the study was much larger than the amount commonly found in supplements. Although large amounts can cause bleeding problems, few people in the study experienced any side effects.

For Alzheimer's sufferers who are only moderately impaired, vitamin E may be just the thing to help them maintain their independence longer.

Raise your glass and lower your risk

A toast to good health! If your glass is filled with wine, your old age may be filled with memories. A recent study conducted in France found that drinking some wine may lower your risk of Alzheimer's.

The study found that among moderate drinkers (people who drank three to four glasses of wine a day) the incidence of Alzheimer's was about 1 percent. About 5 percent of the nondrinkers and mild drinkers developed the disease.

Although moderate alcohol intake may protect against AD, alcoholism contributes to dementia, so don't overdo it. Researchers say there is no reason to advise elderly people who do not drink to start indulging. Also, the people in the study drank only wine, not beer or other alcoholic beverages.

If you don't drink, you shouldn't start in hopes of avoiding Alzheimer's. But if you already drink wine, you may have more reason to toast your good health.

The latest buzz on estrogen and Alzheimer's

Alzheimer's research reveals some bad news for you if you're a woman. You are twice as likely to get Alzheimer's disease as your male counterparts.

Some scientists think women may be more likely to develop Alzheimer's because of the decrease in estrogen levels after menopause. A large study conducted by the National Institute on Aging supports that theory. Researchers found that postmenopausal women who took estrogen were 54 percent less likely to get Alzheimer's than women who had never taken estrogen.

Other studies have found that estrogen may also help ease the symptoms of Alzheimer's — at least short term. In one study, women who already had the disease were treated with estrogen. Within a week, these women showed signs of improvement, while the women who didn't get estrogen did not.

Still, estrogen is a long way from becoming an accepted treatment for Alzheimer's. Other studies have found no benefit to estrogen therapy. In a recent study, researchers gave estrogen to women with mild to moderate Alzheimer's for one year. All of the women in the study had had a hysterectomy. This study found that estrogen made no significant difference in mental functioning.

Obviously, more studies need to be done, and many are underway now. Currently, the bulk of studies suggest that most women would be less likely to develop Alzheimer's if they take estrogen after menopause.

Doctors prescribe estrogen to treat hot flashes and other menopausal symptoms, but future research may find it's more beneficial in preventing serious disorders, like heart disease, osteoporosis, and possibly Alzheimer's.

Despite its healthful possibilities, estrogen is not risk free. It may increase your chances of getting breast cancer and endometrial cancer. You have to weigh the good against the bad, and consider your own risk factors for each of these diseases when deciding whether to take estrogen.

Natural way to 'leaf' AD behind

An herb reputed to improve your memory should help combat a disease that slowly drains your memories out of you, shouldn't it?

According to a new study, it does. Researchers found that an extract made from the nuts, leaves, and branches of the ginkgo biloba tree may slow down the course of Alzheimer's disease for some people. In the study, a substantial number of people with AD who took the extract delayed the progression of the disease by six months to one year.

This effect is about the same as two prescription drugs (Aricept and Cognex) approved by the FDA for treating Alzheimer's. None of the people in the study suffered any significant side effects.

For more information about ginkgo, see the *Memory* chapter.

ANT-i Alzheimer's chemical

Ants can be real pests, especially at picnics, but scientists have put those tiny insects to good use. They've found that a chemical ants give off to help them find their food supply may help slow down the memory loss Alzheimer's causes.

The chemical, anabaseine, is a pheromone that sends a specific message to ant brains. Scientists think it also could benefit humans brains and are studying its usefulness.

Don't rush out to buy an ant farm or throw away your bug spray just yet, though. Scientists say they can make synthetic versions of anabaseine for medicine if it turns out to be helpful.

Simple steps to snuff out Alzheimer's

You know smoking is bad for your lungs, but what does it do to your brain? Earlier studies revealed the surprising conclusion that smoking may protect you against Alzheimer's. These reports were based on the fact that more Alzheimer's victims are nonsmokers.

But a recent study found that smoking actually increases your chances of Alzheimer's and other forms of dementia. More than 6,000 people age 55 and over were followed for two years. Almost 150 people developed Alzheimer's or other dementia during that period. According to researchers, smoking doubled the risk of the disease.

Why the difference in opinion? It may be that nonsmokers live longer and, therefore, have more time to develop the disease. Smoking is the number one cause of premature death in developed countries like the United States. Since Alzheimer's strikes mostly older people, smokers may not be affected simply because they die from lung cancer or other causes before Alzheimer's can develop.

Sewing the seeds of Alzheimer's

You might love your job or hate it, but you should know that your choice of occupations may put you at greater risk of Alzheimer's.

According to researchers, people who have jobs that require tools with electric motors may be more likely to develop AD. These tools can give off electro-magnetic fields (EMFs), which may contribute to the development of the disease.

Seamstresses, dressmakers, and tailors, who work huddled over electric sewing machines, are three times more likely to get Alzheimer's than most people. The only occupations with a greater risk of AD are electric power line workers and welders.

Women in the study who used industrial sewing machines that gave off EMFs were almost four times as likely to get Alzheimer's as women who weren't exposed to EMFs. Recreational use of home sewing machines shouldn't be a problem.

Researchers say industrial electrical equipment can be designed to lessen the danger of exposure to EMFs.

The aluminum connection: Fact or fiction?

You can't live without it. It makes up 60 percent of your body weight, and most people need to drink more of it. And yet, what's in your glass of water may affect whether you will get Alzheimer's as you age.

One of the most controversial risk factors for Alzheimer's is aluminum. You can get it from many sources, including aluminum cookware and antiperspirants, but it is also commonly found in your water supply.

Some studies have found that the brains of people who died from Alzheimer's contained too much aluminum. Does this mean that exposure to aluminum may contribute to AD? Experts still disagree.

One study tested the effect of aluminum, calcium, and fluorine in drinking water on mental function. Researchers also tested the water's pH. According to this study, aluminum in drinking water affected cognitive abilities only when it was found in water with an acid pH.

One good result of the same study was that calcium in drinking water seemed to protect against Alzheimer's.

Most experts don't think aluminum in your drinking water poses a serious threat to your memories. But if you're worried, you can have your water tested, or just buy bottled water. If you also drink a little extra milk, the calcium will help your bones *and* your brain.

Ever hear of this memory thief?

Your daughter says she asked you to pick up your grandson at nursery school this morning. You know your daughter's telling the truth, but you seem to have a black hole where that memory should be. Does this mean you have Alzheimer's?

Don't panic. It may just mean you should have your hearing checked. In a recent, small study, researchers examined some elderly people with memory problems. Almost all of them, 94 percent, also had severe hearing loss. Among healthy elderly people, only about a third have hearing problems.

Researchers don't know if the hearing loss is a symptom or a cause of memory problems. But if you just can't remember recent conversations, have your hearing checked. It might be an easy way to help improve your memory.

Knowledge knocks out Alzheimer's

Education may be the key to success, but it also may be the key to sidestepping Alzheimer's. Recent studies have found that the more education you have, the lower your risk of AD.

Education may protect your brain indirectly by making you more likely to eat better, exercise, and obtain good medical care. However, the most important thing it does is to increase connections between your brain cells.

Alzheimer's disease works by destroying the lines of communication, called synapses, between brain cells. Every time you learn something new, you build new connections, thus strengthening your memory and fighting off AD.

Experts think these connections give you a "cognitive reserve" like money in the bank saved for a rainy day. If you lost your job, that extra money would buy you time before the bank took your home away. In the same way, a large cognitive reserve would give you extra time before the damage from Alzheimer's takes your memories away.

To keep Alzheimer's at bay, try to learn something new every day. A crossword puzzle, word game, picture puzzle, or interesting new book will help get those synapses snapping.

Of course, reading this book is already helping. As you absorb this information, you're building up your cognitive reserve, and you can take that to the bank.

Control your risk with a 'stroke' of luck

Strokes can kill or paralyze you, but new research finds that even small strokes that don't cause such obvious damage can contribute to Alzheimer's.

Researchers found that if you have even one or two small strokes in certain regions of your brain, you may dramatically increase your risk of AD. They studied more than 100 women for the tell-tale lesions of Alzheimer's disease. Among women who had many lesions, those who had the small strokes were more than 20 times as likely to have dementia as women who had never had a stroke.

This may sound like bad news, a double-whammy to your brain delivered by AD and stroke, but it could actually be a stroke of good luck for you. By controlling your risk of stroke, you may lower your risk of losing your mind to Alzheimer's at the same time.

For information about strokes, see the *Stroke* chapter.

Conditions that mimic Alzheimer's

Alzheimer's disease is notorious for mimicking other problems and disorders. That makes it the most overdiagnosed and misdiagnosed disorder of mental functioning in older adults, says the National Institute of Mental Health.

Some potentially treatable conditions that may be mistaken for Alzheimer's include:

- **Side effects of medication.** Some medications or combination of medicines can cause symptoms that seem like Alzheimer's. Taking too much or too little of a prescribed medicine can have the same effect.

- **Toxic substances.** Exposure to toxic substances, like carbon monoxide or methyl alcohol, can create memory loss and other symptoms of Alzheimer's.

- **Circulatory disorders.** Heart disease and strokes may produce problems associated with AD.

- **Infections.** Viral or fungal infections of the brain could cause intellectual, behavioral, or psychological disorders.

- **Trauma.** An injury to your head could cause mental symptoms much later.

- **Substance abuse.** Alcoholism or drug abuse can sometimes cause problems that are mistaken for Alzheimer's.

- **Metabolic disorders.** A malfunctioning thyroid gland, nutritional deficiencies, or anemia can mimic Alzheimer's.

- **Tumors.** Any tumor in your skull can cause pressure that leads to mental symptoms.

- **Neurologic disorders.** Multiple sclerosis, normal-pressure hydrocephalus, and other nervous system disorders can masquerade as symptoms of Alzheimer's.

Other mental disorders, like depression, may also be mistaken for Alzheimer's. Make sure your doctor rules out other possibilities before you accept a diagnosis of Alzheimer's.

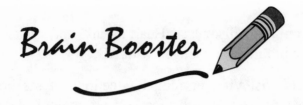

Word search

You can help fend off Alzheimer's by including puzzles in your daily activities. Try this word search and see how many Alzheimer's-related words you can find.

ALUMINUM	ALZHEIMERS
CONFUSION	EDUCATION
ESTROGEN	GINGKO
MEMORIES	MOOD SWINGS
MOTOR SKILLS	NSAIDS
RONALD REAGAN	SPEECH
STROKE	VITAMIN E
WINE	

```
W  G  N  K  N  H  M  U  N  I  M  U  L  A  S
C  I  I  A  S  E  N  I  M  A  T  I  V  D  P
O  F  N  N  G  W  F  E  E  M  G  K  I  J  N
N  J  I  E  G  A  G  U  G  O  M  A  F  L  M
F  S  J  F  O  K  E  E  P  O  S  H  A  I  N
U  E  Z  A  C  Q  O  R  T  N  W  G  N  D  O
S  I  A  Q  E  Q  Q  O  D  F  A  R  G  U  I
I  R  I  C  F  K  R  S  S  L  T  E  O  U  T
O  O  P  Q  O  S  T  D  L  P  A  S  V  Y  A
N  M  R  K  K  R  U  M  S  Y  E  N  P  K  C
X  E  K  I  O  U  J  Q  D  C  X  E  O  P  U
L  M  L  K  J  J  S  Y  C  Y  J  H  C  R  D
Z  L  E  A  A  N  E  G  O  R  T  S  E  H  E
S  O  L  Y  I  S  G  N  I  W  S  D  O  O  M
A  L  Z  H  E  I  M  E  R  S  B  X  Z  X  C
```

Check your answers in the *Solutions to Brain boosters and teasers* section at the back of the book.

Stroke

Preventing and treating a 'brain attack'

Are you ready for some scary numbers? This year, more than half a million Americans will suffer a stroke. Of these, nearly one-third will die, and those who live will probably have some physical or mental damage for the rest of their lives.

Strokes are the third leading cause of death in most industrialized countries. Diabetics, men, smokers, women taking oral contraceptives, and people with high blood pressure or a personal or family history of heart disease or stroke are at high risk of having a stroke.

But the news isn't all bad. By following a healthy lifestyle and knowing the danger signs of stroke, you can greatly reduce your chance of becoming a victim.

Things you should know

A stroke is similar to a heart attack, except it occurs in the brain. That's why some medical experts refer to it as a "brain attack." These are the three major types:

Thrombotic. This is the most common type of stroke. The process begins when fatty deposits called plaques build up in the arteries that supply blood to the brain. This severely reduces the blood flow until, eventually, a clot in an artery entirely blocks the path of blood.

Embolic. An embolic stroke results when a blood clot forms somewhere else in the body, usually in arteries of the heart or neck, and the clot travels through the circulatory system to the brain.

Hemorrhagic. This severe type of stroke is not caused by a blocked blood vessel. It is caused by a blood vessel that leaks blood into the surrounding brain tissue, which can cause brain cell damage. Hemorrhagic strokes can occur for a variety of reasons, but high blood pressure is a factor in many cases.

If the right side of the brain is damaged by a stroke, the victim could be paralyzed on the left side and experience a loss in perception, spacing and memory. If the left side of the brain is damaged, the victim could be paralyzed on the right side and have difficulty with speech and remembering words.

About 10 percent of strokes are preceded by transient ischemic attacks or TIAs. A transient ischemic attack occurs when blood flow is interrupted in some part of the brain for a short period of time, usually without causing long-term damage.

Transient ischemic attacks are sometimes called "little strokes." The symptoms are similar to a stroke, but they last only for a few minutes. People who have experienced one of these temporary blockages of blood flow to the brain are nearly 10 times more likely to suffer a stroke than those who haven't had a TIA.

Warning signs of a stroke

If you experience any of these symptoms, call your doctor and get medical help immediately.

- sudden change in vision, like a flash of blindness, double vision, or dimness of vision, particularly in one eye

- sudden difficulty with speech, including loss of ability to speak or trouble talking or understanding speech

- unexplained or unusually severe headaches or dizziness, especially when associated with other mental or neurological signs

- sudden change in mental abilities

- impaired judgment

- sudden numbness, weakness, or tingling sensations of the face, arm, and leg, usually on one side of the body

- sudden change in personality

- any symptoms, such as paralysis, that seem to occur only on one side of the body

Since 38 percent of all stroke victims die within a month, the 30 days following a stroke are critical. According to the American Heart Association, nearly half the people who survive the first month are still living seven years after their stroke.

How to lower your risk

Most strokes are preventable by eliminating risk factors. The greatest risk factors to beware of are:

High blood pressure. This "silent killer" puts stress on blood vessels and makes circulation more difficult. It may take years for high blood pressure to weaken and damage blood vessels, but a stroke can happen within seconds without warning.

Heart disease. Too much cholesterol can clog your blood vessels and lead to plaque buildup and eventually blocked arteries. Heart disease can also raise your risk of blood clots, another frequent cause of stroke.

Smoking. Tobacco use damages blood vessel walls by weakening them and making them an easier target for an aneurysm. It also tends to harden your arteries, which cuts down on their ability to deliver blood to your brain.

Diabetes. This disease and its complications can raise your risk of stroke if you don't keep it under careful control.

Obesity. Being overweight causes many health problems, including high blood pressure and poor circulation.

If you have any of these risk factors, start to make changes in your diet and lifestyle. Remember — most strokes are preventable.

Beware of Monday mornings

Everybody hates Mondays, and now there's a new reason to mourn the passing of the weekend. According to a research team at the Boston University School of Medicine, more strokes occur on Monday than on any other day of the week.

Other studies have shown similar results. In addition to Mondays, strokes also show a preference for morning hours, with about 35 percent occurring between 8:00 a.m. and noon. The opposite was also true — people were least likely to suffer a stroke between 8:00 p.m. and midnight. Sunday was the lightest stroke day.

Researchers aren't exactly sure why strokes choose Mondays. It could be because many people tend to drink and smoke more on the weekends. The stress of going back to work on Monday morning could also be a factor.

If you are at risk for a stroke, avoid smoking and drinking heavily on the weekends, and learn to reduce your Monday morning stress.

New therapy helps 'rewire' damaged brain

Stroke rehabilitation can be a long and difficult process, and some people never recover completely. Researchers at the University of Alabama, however, have shown that one kind of therapy can actually cause damaged brains to reorganize.

The therapy, called constraint-induced movement therapy (CI therapy), involves tying down a patient's good arm, forcing him to try harder to use the disabled one. The therapy has been very successful, producing improvements even in people who had strokes years before beginning the therapy.

CI therapy is believed to work by forcing nearby brain cells to take over for the damaged ones. The new study used a brain-mapping technique called focal transcranial magnetic stimulation to see if this was actually the case.

The researchers were excited that the study participants showed immediate improvements when they began therapy. And six months later, they had maintained those improvements.

The brain mapping also showed changes in the surface of the brain as soon as therapy began. By the end of the first day, the stroke-damaged part of the brain had almost twice as many active areas. Six months after treatment, brain activity was about equal in both sides of the brain — the stroke-damaged side and the unaffected side.

This research provides exciting evidence that the brain can recover after stroke, and it may lead to even more effective therapies.

Another reason to quit smoking

Smokers are twice as likely as nonsmokers to suffer a stroke, and for those who smoke more than a pack a day, the numbers go even higher.

A recent study that followed 22,000 male smokers for over a decade showed that smoking caused a greater number of strokes, even in people who were otherwise in perfect health. A similar, 12-year study of 117,000 female smokers showed that the risk of stroke continues to go up with each extra cigarette smoked each day.

The good news about smoking is that quitting lowers your risk of stroke. The same studies that showed the increase in stroke among smokers also showed this — after a few years, people who quit smoking were at the same risk levels as people who never smoked. For women, the increased risk was almost totally gone within two to four years of quitting.

Exercise — but don't overdo it

Exercise is one of the basic building blocks of good health, but more is not always better. In fact, when it comes to stroke, exercise can only lower your risk so far, according to a Harvard report.

In a 20-year study of 11,000 men, researchers found that burning between 1,000 and 3,000 calories per week did indeed lower stroke risk. But working out harder and longer did not lower the risk any further. The study also shows that in order to be effective, exercise needs to be at least moderately strenuous — walking instead of bowling, for instance.

You can easily burn 1,000 calories by walking briskly for 30 minutes five or six times a week. Or, if you'd like some company, grab a partner for a game of tennis or an evening of dancing. You'll both reap the benefits of stroke protection.

Why you need to get rid of anger

Need another reason to relax? Researchers in the United States and Japan say anger and aggression can raise your risk of stroke.

After evaluating people's personalities, researchers used ultrasound technology to measure the amount of blockage in the carotid arteries, which carry blood to the head and neck. They found that over half of the people with severe blockages rated very high on the anger scale, while only 16 percent of more relaxed people had severe blockages.

These findings support earlier studies that proved the same thing for heart disease, high blood pressure, and other health problems. While they aren't sure whether anger causes the blockage or the blockage causes anger, the link between the two conditions is obvious. Many doctors also think stress can damage the brain's arteries.

If you can't find a way to relax on your own, seek professional help. Taking a few training sessions in anger control or stress management could make all the difference in your risk of heart attack and stroke.

Discover the power of milk

Strong teeth and strong bones aren't the only reasons to drink milk. Researchers say the more milk you drink, the less likely you are to suffer a stroke. In fact, people who don't drink milk have double the stroke rate of people who drink at least 16 ounces every day.

Researchers aren't sure why milk has this effect, since calcium from nondairy sources does not produce the same result. It could mean that milk has an unidentified ingredient that helps prevent stroke. Or maybe the milk drinkers in the study group were just more health conscious overall.

Drinking four cups a day will satisfy your daily calcium requirements, and it might fortify your body against strokes as well.

Aspirin controversy — what should you do?

Taking aspirin every day may be sound advice for protecting your heart, but it might not be good for your brain.

Researchers at Johns Hopkins and Tulane universities analyzed 16 studies involving people who had suffered hemorrhagic strokes. This type of stroke occurs when a weakened artery in your brain bursts. They found that although aspirin makes you less likely to have a heart attack or ischemic stroke, it may increase your risk of having a hemorrhagic stroke.

The researchers concluded that the benefits of aspirin therapy for your heart probably outweigh the danger in stroke risk. But this may not be true for all people. If you are at high risk for hemorrhagic stroke, talk with your doctor before starting an aspirin-a-day routine.

'Good' cholesterol keeps arteries clean

If you have heart disease, you also have a greater chance of suffering a stroke. The fatty deposits in the blood vessels around your heart are the same kind that build up in the carotid arteries in your neck, blocking the flow of blood and oxygen to your brain.

A recent study has shown that among men with heart disease, the greatest risk of stroke wasn't found in those with abnormally high total cholesterol levels, or those with huge amounts of bad LDL cholesterol. Instead, the danger was greatest for those with low levels of good HDL cholesterol. That's because HDLs carry cholesterol away from the arteries to the liver, where it is broken down and disposed of.

In the study, more than 80 percent of the men with low HDL had already developed carotid atherosclerosis, blockages of fatty plaque in the large arteries of the neck. Carotid atherosclerosis increases your stroke risk by 20 to 40 percent.

Ask your doctor about your cholesterol levels. If your HDL cholesterol level is too low, you can raise it by exercising regularly and maintaining a healthy weight.

Researchers say women have fewer strokes

Tired of taking your hormone replacement therapy? Well, it might be a good idea to stick with it. Doctors are now saying that higher levels of estrogen in the blood may be the reason women don't have strokes as often as men. And when a woman does have a stroke, estrogen might play a key role in limiting the damage.

Researchers at the famous Johns Hopkins Medical School believe the results of their animal tests will soon be vitally important to stroke prevention in humans. Their research proved that female rats have a greater flow of blood to the brain than male rats. This greater flow stops the brain from suffering as much damage during a stroke. However, when they took out the female rats' ovaries beforehand, the amount of brain damage from the stroke went up to the level of the males.

Similar trends have been shown in humans. Premenopausal women, as a rule, suffer much less brain damage after a stroke than men who are the same age. After menopause, when there is less estrogen in a woman's bloodstream, both stroke risk and stroke damage rise dramatically.

More tests are on the way to determine if giving estrogen to people suffering a stroke would help prevent brain damage afterward. There are also ongoing efforts to find a way to apply this estrogen benefit to men.

New hope for stroke victims

If you think you are having a stroke, call for help and get to the hospital as quickly as possible — every second counts. Special procedures and treatments can limit the damage, but the longer you wait, the less likely they are to be effective.

New treatments are always being developed, such as an enzyme shot that is designed to go right to the problem. Doctors at a hospital in Oregon recently used this amazing new therapy to bring back a stroke victim who had lost all brain activity. By injecting the enzyme directly into his brain arteries, the doctors were able to dissolve the clot that was cutting off oxygen and save him, even though he had suffered a stroke more than nine hours before.

"Life shrinks or expands in proportion to one's courage."
— Anais Nin

Healing your brain after a stroke

The severity of a stroke can range from a mild, momentary lapse of oxygen to a massive blockage that causes severe damage. Regardless of the severity, the road to recovery can be frustrating, and the sooner you get started, the better.

Walking. Your recovery will most likely involve physical therapy to improve your balance and coordination. Stretching and various other exercises will help to restore your muscle tone and general fitness, particularly if you have paralysis.

Talking. After a stroke, speaking can become awkward. You may have trouble finding the right word or difficulty putting together the pieces of a sentence. Speech therapy can help improve your speaking and language skills.

Self-reliance. Occupational therapy can help you re-learn the skills you need to care for yourself. Everyday tasks, like bathing and cooking, that were simple before the stroke can seem like impossible challenges afterward. Regaining the ability to look after yourself is an important part of your physical recovery, and it also plays an enormous part in your emotional healing.

Coping. Special counseling for your family and friends can help them cope with the aftereffects of your stroke. They will also learn how to help you help yourself.

Remember, patience and dedication are the keys to your recovery. Everyone moves at a different pace — be determined, not rushed. The degree of your commitment is closely linked to the degree of your success.

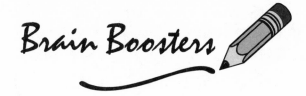

High-ho

Have a "high" old time identifying words and phrases that contain the word "high" from the clues below.

1. An infant's throne _ _ _ _ _ _ _ _ _

2. No matter what _ _ _ _ _ _ _ _ _ _ _ _ _ _ _ _ _ _ _

3. Hit the road _ _ _ _ _ _ _ _

4. Gary Cooper's time of day _ _ _ _ _ _ _ _

5. Above the drumstick _ _ _ _ _ _

6. They go with pantyhose _ _ _ _ _ _ _ _ _

7. Congratulate by slapping _ _ _ _ _ _ _ _

8. Lively pranks _ _ _ _ _ _ _ _ _

9. Outstanding part _ _ _ _ _ _ _ _ _

10. To a grasshopper (very small) _ _ _ _ _ _ _ _

Check your answers in the *Solutions to Brain boosters and teasers* section at the back of the book.

What's the difference?

Look closely at both of these drawings. Can you find 10 ways the second drawing is different from the first?

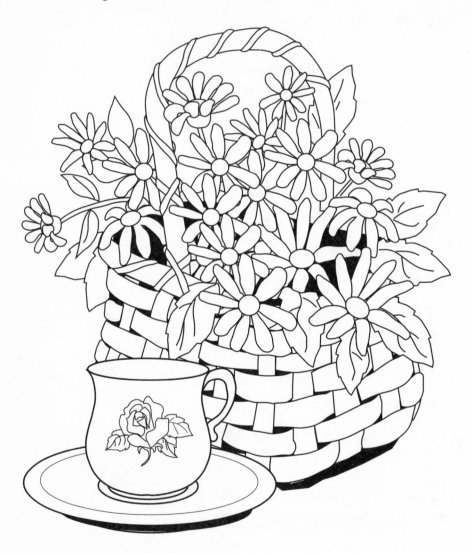

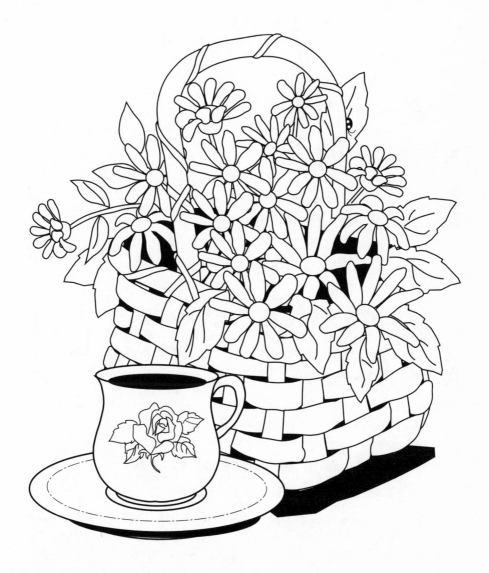

Check your answers in the *Solutions to Brain boosters and teasers* section at the back of the book.

Nutrition

Food for thought

The next time you can't remember how to spell "pneumonia" or struggle to balance your checkbook, take a look at what you eat everyday. Experts say eating certain foods can help keep your brain in tiptop shape, while others might be harmful.

Soy linked to higher rates of senility

If you've started eating tofu burgers instead of hamburgers because you think soy is healthier — you may be in for a surprise. New research suggests that eating tofu may make your brain age faster, leading to serious problems with memory and learning in later years.

Even if you never eat tofu — a custard-like food made from pureed soybeans — you're still not in the clear. Soy or soybean oil can be found in everything from salad dressings, mayonnaise, and margarine to breakfast cereals and energy bars, making it the most widely used oil. It is estimated that soy protein is in 60 percent of all processed foods. And soy protein is added to the food of cattle and other livestock, so you may consume it indirectly just by eating your usual steak or hamburger.

Researchers in Hawaii concluded that soy may contribute to brain aging after examining the diets of more than 8,000 Japanese-American men for over 30 years. They found that those who ate two or more servings of tofu a week were much more likely to become senile or forgetful as they grew older compared with men who ate little or no tofu.

The more tofu the subjects ate, the more learning and memory problems they suffered in later life. Loss of mental function occurred in 4 percent of the men who ate the least amount of tofu compared with 19 percent of the men who ate the greatest amount of tofu.

These are shocking results for a food that has been touted for its health benefits and was recently given FDA approval to make health claims on package labels.

Dr. Lon White, lead researcher of the Hawaiian study, suggests the study's findings should make people think twice about the amount of soy they eat. "What we have here is a scary idea that may turn out to be dead wrong," he says. "Or it could turn out to be the first uncovering of an important health-negative effect of a food that we believe may have a lot of good going for it."

White's study, which began in 1965, included subjects ranging from 46 to 65 years old. The men were asked whether they ate certain foods associated with a traditional Japanese diet or an American diet. They were interviewed about their dietary habits again in the early 1970s and were tested for cognitive function — including attention, concentration, memory, language skills, and judgment — in the early 1990s when they were 71 to 93 years old. They were also given a brain scan at that time.

The results were disturbing. Out of 26 foods studied, only tofu was found to be significantly related to brain function. Men who had a high intake of tofu not only scored lower on tests of mental ability, but their brains were more likely to show signs of advanced age and shrinkage. Their test scores were typical of a person four years older.

Although the study was done on men, researchers also interviewed and tested 502 wives of the men in the study — and came up with similar findings.

The study has created a stir because it contradicts previous research that has found soy to be beneficial. Earlier studies have shown that soy may fight cancer and heart disease, prevent osteoporosis, and relieve menopause symptoms. Researchers credit estrogen-like molecules called isoflavones for soy's apparent disease-fighting properties. But those same substances could have negative effects on the body as well, White notes. He says people need to understand that isoflavones are complex chemicals that act like drugs and change the body's chemistry.

"The great things they [consumers] have been hearing about soy foods in recent years have little to do with nutrients — carbohydrates, proteins, fats, minerals, vitamins," he says. "All that hype is related to the idea that soy contains other kinds of molecules that act like medicines ... they alter the way our body chemistry works."

The isoflavones in soy are a type of phytoestrogen or plant estrogen, which mimics the estrogen produced naturally in your body. Brain cells have receptors that link up with estrogen to help maintain brain function, and White speculates that phytoestrogens may compete with the body's natural estrogens for these receptors.

Soy's isoflavones are also thought to interfere with enzymes and amino acids in the brain. One of soy's main isoflavones, genistein, has been shown to limit the enzyme tyrosine kinase in the hippocampus — the brain's memory center. By interfering with the activity of this enzyme, genistein blocks a process called "long-term potentiation" that is central to learning and memory.

Dr. Larrian Gillespie, author of *The Menopause Diet*, says eating too much soy could result in other problems as well. She has found that consuming 40 milligrams (mg) of isoflavones a day can slow down thyroid function, resulting in hypothyroidism. Most isoflavone supplements come in a 40-mg dose, and just 6 ounces of tofu or 2 cups of soy milk would supply the same amount.

Also, because isoflavones act like estrogen, some studies suggest that postmenopausal women who eat a lot of soy may increase their risk of breast cancer. And scientists have questioned the potential effects of soy on infants as well. One study found that infants who drank soy formula received six to 11 times as many phytoestrogens as the amount known to have hormonal effects in adults. Some think this could lead to early puberty, which is associated with a greater risk for breast cancer and ovarian cysts.

This leads to the question of whether soy's good aspects outweigh the negative ones.

"Whatever good effects come with the gift [soy], will also come at some cost," White says. "We do not know yet just what those costs are, just as we really don't know yet the full and honest extent of their health benefits. We're flying blind … and my data … are very, very disturbing."

The Hawaiian study was a long-term, well-designed, controlled study, but it was just one study. The results are strong enough to make everyone sit up and take notice, but more research needs to be done to confirm the results. If you eat soy, you may want to err on the side of caution. Be sure you know the amount of soy isoflavones you consume each day, and steer clear of soy supplements and soy-enriched foods (like some nutritional bars) until more research is done.

The following chart will help you determine the isoflavone content of some common soy products.

How many soy isoflavones do you consume?

Food	Milligrams of isoflavones *	Serving size (approximate)
Bacon, meatless	1.9	2 strips (1/2 ounce)
Granola bar (hard, plain)	.1	3.5 ounce
Harvest Burger, (all vegetable protein patty)	8.2	1 patty
Infant formula, Prosobee® and Isomil® with iron, ready-to-feed	8	1 cup
Miso	43	1/2 cup
Peanuts, raw	.3	1/2 cup
Soy breakfast links (45 g)	1.7	2 links
Soy cheese, cheddar	7	3.5 ounce
Soy flour (textured)	148	1/2 cup
Soy hot dog (51 g)	3	2 hot dogs
Soy milk	20	1 cup
Soy powder (vanilla shake)	14 – 42 **	1 scoop
Soy protein nutritional bar	14 – 42 **	1 bar
Soy sauce, made from hydrolyzed vegetable protein	.1	1/2 cup
Soy sauce, made from soy and wheat	1.6	1/2 cup
Soybean chips	54	1/2 cup
Soybeans (roasted)	128	1/2 cup
Tempeh	44	1/2 cup
Tofu (silken, firm)	28	1/2 cup
Tofu, yogurt	16	1/2 cup
USDA Commodity, beef patties with Vegetable Protein Product (VPP), frozen, cooked®	1.9	3.5 ounces

* Data from USDA – Iowa State University Database on the Isoflavone Content of Food – 1999.

** Data derived from Protein Technologies International.

® VPP is often used in school lunch programs.

Powerful protection from tea

Green and black teas contain powerful antioxidants called polyphenols. In fact, five cups of tea a day can give you as much antioxidant protection as two servings of veggies. So sit back, relax, and sip something good for you.

Unleash the power of fruits and veggies

Your brain is a real oxygen hog. Although it makes up only a small percentage of your body weight, it uses about 20 percent of the oxygen you inhale.

You couldn't live without oxygen, but as your body processes this essential gas, it sometimes creates harmful, unstable molecules called free radicals. Since your brain uses so much oxygen, it may be a particular target for free radical damage.

Luckily, your body produces natural free radical scavengers called antioxidants. You can also get them from food. Colorful fruits and vegetables are rich in antioxidants. The brighter and deeper the color, the more antioxidant power contained inside. Vitamin C, vitamin E, beta carotene, selenium, and zinc are powerful antioxidants.

The U.S. Department of Agriculture recommends that you eat at least five servings of fruits and vegetables every day. Here are five simple ways to get your five a day.

- Keep a bag of baby carrots in your refrigerator for a quick and easy snack.

- Add more vegetables to your sandwiches. Instead of just the usual lettuce and tomato, add some cucumber slices, diced carrots, or green and red pepper strips.

- To save time, buy pre-packaged salads at the grocery store.

- Slice a banana into your cereal and have a glass of juice.

- Although fresh is usually better, don't count out canned or frozen fruits and vegetables. They're convenient and their nutritional value is close to fresh.

With just a little effort, you can get your five daily servings of healthful fruits and veggies. If you're not sure what counts as a serving, here are some examples.

Vegetables	Fruits
1/2 cup cooked or canned vegetables	a whole fruit (medium apple, pear, banana, or orange)
1 cup raw leafy vegetables (a small salad)	a grapefruit half
6 to 8 carrot sticks (3-inches long)	a melon wedge
1 medium potato	1/4 cup dried fruit
3/4 cup vegetable juice	1/2 cup berries
1/2 cup cooked or canned dry beans or peas	3/4 cup fruit juice

You are what you eat

Are you feeling a little down? Would you feel better if you had a pint of Ben and Jerry's in front of you? Researchers say there is a connection between what you eat and how you feel, and here's why.

Your brain uses chemical messengers called neurotransmitters to move information between brain cells. Some of these chemicals also help you feel happier, calmer, more relaxed, energetic, or alert. Certain foods can boost or suppress the amount of neurotransmitters in your brain.

The most well-known neurotransmitter is serotonin. Serotonin helps regulate your appetite and your sleep cycle and is associated with a peaceful, relaxed feeling. Most antidepressant medications work by increasing the amount of serotonin circulating in your brain.

When your brain is low in serotonin, your body craves carbohydrates, like sugar, bread, and pasta. These foods raise your serotonin level.

Serotonin is made from tryptophan, an essential amino acid that comes from protein-rich foods, like turkey, dairy products, and nuts. When you eat these foods, tryptophan gets into your blood. To move the tryptophan into your brain, you need carbohydrates.

This could explain why snacking on a candy bar may raise your mood temporarily — but only if you've already eaten enough protein to get some tryptophan into your bloodstream.

But don't overdo it. Too much protein has the opposite effect — other amino acids compete with tryptophan for absorption into your brain.

The Recommended Dietary Allowance (RDA) for protein is 63 grams for men ages 25 and over. For women ages 25 and over, the RDA is 50 grams.

Vegetables from the sea

Seaweed for brain power? Sure. Seaweed, algae, kelp, and phytoplankton make up the undersea vegetarian diet of many fish. It's from these plants that fish build up their stores of omega-3 and other fatty acids.

So if you're looking for a unique path to better thinking, or if you're just not hungry for fish, order some seaweed at a Japanese restaurant. It might be the "smartest" decision you've ever made.

Turn back the clock with these vitamins

You don't have to be malnourished to feel the effects of a vitamin deficiency. Even a small vitamin deficiency can dull your mental abilities.

Vitamin E. One of the most exciting discoveries in Alzheimer's research was finding that vitamin E may help prevent or treat this memory-robbing disease. This powerful antioxidant may also work to protect your brain from free radical damage. Good food sources include wheat germ, soybeans, mangoes, almonds, sunflower seeds, wheat germ oil, canola oil, and safflower oil. You can also buy supplements.

The Recommended Dietary Allowance for vitamin E is 15 International Units (IU) or 10 milligrams (mg) for men and 12 IU or 8 mg for women. Most studies used a much higher dosage, as much as 2,000 IU daily.

Although vitamin E is relatively safe, large doses over 400 IU taken over a prolonged period of time may cause nausea, intestinal discomfort, dizziness, headaches, or unusual fatigue.

Ask your doctor's advice before taking vitamin E supplements, especially if you have any health problem or if you are taking blood thinning medication.

Vitamin C. Studies find that low blood levels of vitamin C can impair your memory and mental abilities. You can get enough of this vitamin by eating citrus fruits, like oranges and grapefruit. Other food sources include broccoli, green and red peppers, cantaloupe, and strawberries.

B complex vitamins. Although the B vitamins are separate substances, they often work together. It is very unusual to have a deficiency of just one B vitamin.

- **Thiamin.** Not getting enough thiamin interferes with your brain's ability to use glucose, its major energy source. You can get thiamin by eating nuts, beans, whole grain products, and brown rice.

- **Folic acid.** This important B vitamin helps maintain serotonin levels in your brain. A folic acid deficiency can cause depression or other mental disorders. Food sources include liver, beans, and green leafy vegetables, like spinach.

- **Vitamin B6 (pyridoxine).** A deficiency of B6 interferes with your brain's ability to make neurotransmitters and can lead to depression, shortened attention span, and other mental problems. Bananas, sweet potatoes, baked potatoes, cooked spinach, chicken, and beef liver are rich in vitamin B6.

- **Niacin.** Memory loss is a major symptom of niacin deficiency. Your body can make niacin from tryptophan, an amino acid also important to your brain's health. To get your niacin naturally, eat tuna, liver, chicken, beef, enriched cereals, baked potatoes, and mushrooms.

- **Vitamin B12 (cobalamin).** An estimated 80 to 90 percent of people with a B12 deficiency will develop a nervous system disorder. This vitamin helps your body manufacture neurotransmitters. Without enough vitamin B12, you could suffer memory loss, depression, or other mood disorders. Vitamin B12 is only found in foods from animal origins. Strict vegetarians may need to take supplements. Good sources include beef, chicken livers, dairy products, and fish.

Maximize your mind with minerals

Your body needs only small amounts of most minerals, but don't mistake small for unimportant. They contribute greatly to the health of your bones, blood, and organs, including your brain. You simply couldn't live without them.

Boron. This trace mineral has not yet been recognized as an essential nutrient, but it may be essential to your brain. Studies show that low levels of dietary boron result in poorer performance on tests of eye-hand coordination, long-term and short-term memory, perception, and manual dexterity. Boron also helps your body absorb calcium, so it's important for strong bones. Good food sources include leafy vegetables, soybeans, apples, raisins, almonds, Brazil nuts, and grains.

Zinc. This essential mineral plays multiple roles in your body, but it may be especially important to your brain. Research finds that a deficiency of zinc can cause problems with learning, memory, and attention span. One study even found that too little zinc, paired with an excess of copper, may contribute to violent behavior. Zinc is also important for maintaining sharp senses, including sight, smell, and taste. Oysters are the richest source of zinc, but you can also get it from meat, dairy products, whole grains, eggs, and legumes, like peanuts and lima beans.

Iron. A deficiency of iron can result in anemia, which causes symptoms like apathy, listlessness, clumsiness, irritability, learning disorders, lowered IQ, and shortened attention span. The richest dietary source of iron is liver, but if you just can't stand liver, eat more leafy green vegetables, whole grains, raisins, beans, and molasses.

Copper. Copper helps your body absorb iron. You only need a small amount, which is easy to get from food. Organ meats, seafood, nuts, and seeds are good sources. A copper deficiency is very rare. Supplements are not recommended because too much copper can cause serious mental problems.

Sure-fire way to start your day

Are you a breakfast skipper? If you want to improve your brain, eat breakfast, even if it means grabbing a bagel on the go.

Good nutrition contributes to a better mind, but timing also plays a part. By the time you wake up in the morning, your body has gone about 12 hours without fuel. You may feel fine at first, but by midmorning, your brain may begin to sputter, like a car running out of gas. Starting off your day with a nutritious breakfast will make your mind sharper.

In one study, researchers found that kids who ate a breakfast of sugared corn flakes and a glass of whole milk at school, and then were tested shortly afterward, scored much higher than the kids who had skipped breakfast.

The researchers say it's possible sugar in the breakfast also had something to do with the increase in performance. That's because several studies show that sugar might temporarily boost brain power.

In a recent study, researchers gave lemonade sweetened with either sugar or an artificial sweetener to the study participants, and then tested their memories. The people who got the sugar-sweetened lemonade did better on the tests than the people who got lemonade with the artificial sweetener saccharine. And the positive effects of the sugar lasted into the next day.

Since glucose is the main fuel your brain uses for energy, these results shouldn't be surprising. The key to boosting your brain power seems to be stable blood sugar levels, which means huge amounts of sugar won't help.

Experts say the best way to keep your blood sugar level steady is by eating several small meals throughout the day, instead of three big meals.

Natural way to spice up your memory

Whether you grow them in your garden or buy them in a health food store, herbs are definitely hot items these days. They not only brighten your garden and flavor your food, they may help keep your brain healthy.

Ginkgo. Studies show that extracts of the ginkgo tree can increase blood flow to the brain. More blood flow means more brain power and better short-term memory. And, the older you are, the better ginkgo seems to work. One study found that blood flow to the brain was increased by about 20 percent for people ages 30 to 50, but for people ages 50 to 70, the increase was 70 percent.

Ginseng. This root may help improve your memory and concentration. In one study, researchers found that radio operators given ginseng extract transmitted text faster and made fewer mistakes than operators who did not take ginseng. It may also help lessen stress and increase energy.

St. John's wort. This brightly flowered plant can help brighten your mood. Researchers find that St. John's wort is effective in relieving depression, which can affect concentration, memory, and decision making.

Valerian. This herb acts as a mild sedative. It helps you sleep better at night so you can think clearer during the day.

Beware of these dangerous herbs

While many herbs provide natural ways to improve your health, some herbs can cause dangerous side effects.

- **Chaparral.** Used as a cure for acne and for stopping the aging process, this supplement can cause liver disease.

- **Comfrey.** Speeds healing and prevents bruises and swelling from injuries when used in a paste. Don't take it by mouth because it contains alkaloids that might cause cancer.

- **Ephedra.** Also known as ma-huang, this herb is sold as an energy booster, mood enhancer, and weight loss aid. Serious side effects, including sudden death, heart attack, stroke, chest pain, dizziness, headache, nausea, vomiting, and seizure, have been reported.

- **Germander.** Germander is used to fight obesity, but it may cause hepatitis, an inflammation of the liver.

- **Pokeroot.** Extremely toxic. Side effects include diarrhea, vomiting, and low blood pressure.

- **Sassafras.** Contains safrole, which has been proven to cause cancer.

- **Mistletoe.** Although a pharmaceutical version of mistletoe has been patented, home use is not recommended. The berries are poisonous, and the leaves may cause dangerous blood pressure problems.

Why you might need chocolate

It's two in the afternoon, and you're craving chocolate. As you sink your teeth into a chewy fudge brownie, you wonder if there's something in chocolate that stirs these cravings. Some researchers think so.

One study found that chocolate contains substances that act on your brain the same way cannabinoids do. Cannabinoids come from plant-based drugs and are associated with an elevation in mood and sensitivity.

Chocolate also contains the amino acid phenylalanine, which your body uses to make tyrosine, another amino acid. Tyrosine forms part of epinephrine and norepinephrine, chemical messengers that relay messages from your nervous system throughout your body. The sugar in chocolate may also increase serotonin levels in your brain, which can help you feel relaxed and peaceful.

Wake up your brain cells with coffee

When you get up in the morning, do you stumble straight to your coffeepot? If you feel like your brain is full of fog until you drink at least one cup of coffee, you may be right.

Caffeine helps wake up your brain cells and increase your attentiveness by blocking adenosine, a neurotransmitter that calms your brain.

A recent study found that caffeine may also be an effective pain reliever. People in the study who were given caffeine had less muscle pain after exercise than those who didn't have caffeine. Researchers think adenosine may play a role in causing muscle pain. By blocking adenosine, caffeine could help relieve pain.

Despite the benefits, too much caffeine can cause anxiety, insomnia, headaches, upset stomach, and panic attacks. One or two cups a day should be enough to perk up your mental performance.

The latest buzz on fad diets

Dieting is a way of life for many people. Diet books and quick weight loss products crowd store shelves. And for good reason. An estimated 58 million Americans are overweight, which contributes to many health problems, including diabetes and heart disease.

Instead of following a sensible eating and exercise plan, many people resort to fad diets or diet pills. This can have severe consequences for your brain.

Many popular fad diets emphasize eating one type of food at the expense of balanced nutrition. For example, a diet that contains almost no carbohydrates can result in dehydration and electrolyte imbalance. A diet deficient in protein can result in lack of energy and irritability. It can also cause your body to draw protein from your muscles. Any diet that doesn't include a variety of food can also result in vitamin and mineral deficiencies.

People who follow a very low calorie diet run the risk of permanently damaging their bodies. They also increase their risk of developing an eating disorder, like anorexia. Anorexics severely limit their food intake, resulting in extreme weight loss and, possibly, brain shrinkage. According to a recent study, this shrinkage is not corrected after recovery from the disorder. That means the mind-draining effects may be permanent.

Severely overweight people may be helped by diet pills, taken under a doctor's supervision. The diet pill combination of phentermine and fenfluramine (fen/phen) was taken off the market because of reports that it caused serious heart abnormalities. According to the National Institute of Mental Health, the use of fenfluramine may have also caused irreversible loss of serotonin nerve terminals in some people. This could result in anxiety, depression, and memory problems.

Although being overweight increases your risk of many serious health problems, be wise about your diet choices.

Easy-to-follow nutrition-packed menu

Wondering what to eat for a day's worth of healthful, brain-boosting nutrition? Just turn the page.

When	What	Why
Breakfast	One cup of whole grain cereal or one slice of whole wheat toast, one cup of low-fat milk or 8 ounces of low-fat yogurt, one banana or one-half grapefruit, and one cup of orange juice or cranberry juice	A balanced breakfast starts your day off right. Have some carbohydrates (cereal or toast) and some protein (milk or yogurt). Fruit gives you vitamins and free radical fighting antioxidants.
Midmorning snack	Raisins or low-fat yogurt with fruit or one boiled egg and whole wheat crackers or one bagel	Keep your sugar level on an even keel with healthful snacks, like fruit with a little protein, such as yogurt or an egg.
Lunch	Tuna fish or roast beef sandwich on whole wheat bread, one tossed salad with low-fat dressing, or one cup of vegetable soup and one piece of fresh fruit	Tuna provides brain-boosting omega-3s, and fresh fruits and veggies supply antioxidant power.
Afternoon snack	Baby carrots or celery sticks and 1 ounce of low-fat cheese or cottage cheese	Carrots are high in beta-carotene, and cheese provides calcium and protein.
Dinner	4 ounces broiled salmon or 6 ounces grilled chicken breast, one cup of green beans or broccoli, one baked potato or sweet potato, one tossed salad with low-fat dressing, and one cup of low-fat milk	Make sure you fulfill your five-to-nine servings of fruits and vegetables for the day.
Evening snack	Air-popped popcorn or 1 ounce peanuts	A light snack of complex carbohydrates will help you wind down.

Throughout the day, be sure to drink at least 8 glasses of water. Water transports nutrients throughout your body. Without it, all the other nutrients would be useless.

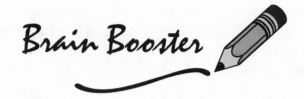

Find the foods

1. APRICOT. The pit of this fruit was used to make the controversial cancer drug, Laetrile.

2. AVOCADO. The highest calorie fruit.

3. BANANA. The most-often eaten fruit in the United States.

4. CHEESE. Blue-veined, soft, or hard-pressed.

5. DARK. Type of turkey meat that contains the most calories.

6. ORCHID. Plant that natural vanilla flavoring is made from.

7. RICE. This food grows in paddies.

8. RIPEN. What a pineapple doesn't do after it's picked.

9. SACCHARIN. It is 550 times sweeter than sugar.

10. SALT. The most commonly used seasoning in the world.

11. SEEDS. What navel oranges don't have.

12. TOMATOES. Love apples.

13. WATER. What is inside a popcorn kernel that makes it pop.

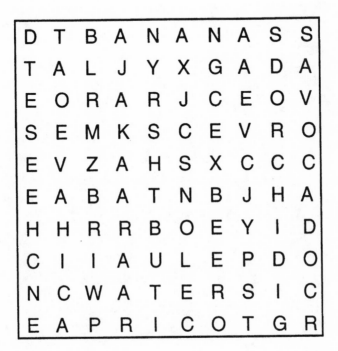

```
D  T  B  A  N  A  N  A  S  S
T  A  L  J  Y  X  G  A  D  A
E  O  R  A  R  J  C  E  O  V
S  E  M  K  S  C  E  V  R  O
E  V  Z  A  H  S  X  C  C  C
E  A  B  A  T  N  B  J  H  A
H  H  R  R  B  O  E  Y  I  D
C  I  I  A  U  L  E  P  D  O
N  C  W  A  T  E  R  S  I  C
E  A  P  R  I  C  O  T  G  R
```

Check your answers in the *Solutions to Brain boosters and teasers* section at the back of the book.

Solutions to Brain boosters and teasers

Cranial crossword solution, page 16

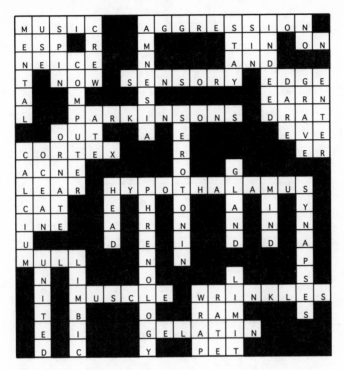

Know your body, page 28

1. Your skin.
2. Your ear.
3. Your tongue.
4. Your hearing.
5. Because its scientific name is the humerus.
6. At the base of your spine. It is a small bone.
7. At the base of your fingernails and toenails.
8. Your hearing.
9. Whiskers.
10. Smell.
11. The gluteus maximus, located in your buttocks.
12. A sneeze.
13. Sweet, sour, bitter, and salty.
14. Your brain.
15. Your eyes.
16. The uvula.
17. The clavicle, or collarbone.
18. Your sense of smell.
19. Your eyes.
20. 206.

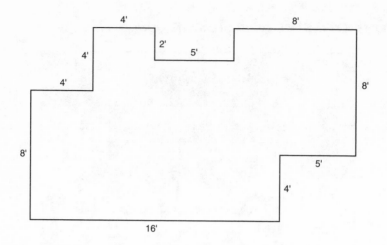

His and hers, page 35

Answers:

Question 1: 7 yards
Question 2: $560

The width of the room at the widest places is 12 feet (8' + 4'), the same as the width of the carpet roll. The length, when measured across the widest part, measures 21 feet (16' + 5'). To convert that to yards, divide by three (1 yard = 3 feet), and you get 7 yards.

To figure the cost:

Width: 12 feet = 4 yards (12 divided by 3)   Length: 7 yards
4 x 7 = 28 square yards

$20 x 28 = $ 560

(You'll be able to lay it in one piece by removing a 2'x 5', a 4'x 4', and a 5'x 4' section.)

Word maker, page 36

improve	improvise	mire	miser	moire
mope	more	move	mover	movie
over	perm	pier	pore	pose
poser	prime	prism	prom	prove
rime	ripe	rise	rope	romp
rose	rove	semi	simper	sire
some	sore	sperm	spire	spore
viper	vise	visor		

'A' is for alphabet, page 53

1. 7 W of the A W = Seven Wonders of the Ancient World
2. 1,001 A N = 1,001 Arabian Nights
3. 12 S of the Z = 12 Signs of the Zodiac
4. 54 C in a D (with the Js) = 54 Cards in a Deck (with the Jokers)
5. 9 P in the S S = 9 Planets in the Solar System
6. 88 P K = 88 Piano Keys
7. 13 S on the A F = 13 Stripes on the American Flag
8. 32 D F at which W F = 32 Degrees Fahrenheit at which Water Freezes
9. 18 H on a G C = 18 Holes on a Golf Course
10. 90 D in a R A = 90 Degrees in a Right Angle
11. 200 D for P G in M = 200 Dollars for Passing Go in Monopoly
12. 8 S on a S S = 8 Sides on a Stop Sign
13. 3 B M (S H T R) = 3 Blind Mice (See How They Run)
14. 4 Q in a G = 4 Quarts in a Gallon
15. 24 H in a D = 24 Hours in a Day
16. 1 W on a U = 1 Wheel on a Unicycle
17. 5 D in a Z C = 5 Digits in a Zip Code
18. 57 H V = 57 Heinz Varieties
19. 11 P on a F T = 11 Players on a Football Team
20. 1,000 W that a P is W = 1,000 Words that a Picture is Worth
21. 29 D in F in a L Y = 29 Days in February in a Leap Year
22. 64 S on a C = 64 Squares on a Checkerboard
23. 40 D and N of the G F = 40 Days and Nights of the Great Flood

Memory checkup, pages 74-75

A total score of	means your memory is
27 - 58	generally good
59 - 116	average
117 - 243	below average

If you scored below average, don't worry. Your life may just be busier than most people, giving you more opportunities to forget things. In an informal survey using this test, the people who scored the poorest tended to be mothers with more than one child living at home. The more things you need to remember — lunch money, laundry, errands, etc. — the more likely you are to forget a few things.

Putting your skills to work, pages 81, 85, & 94

Friday. Friday was the name of the man's horse. This puzzle is a good example of the simple solution that hides just around the corner and is camouflaged by the fact that people have a hard time separating themselves from their first impression. When you hear "Friday," you think "day of the week." But in this case, that's wrong.

The coal, carrot and scarf. These are the remains of a melted snowman. The five pieces of coal were the snowman's buttons and eyes, the carrot was his nose, and the scarf was around his neck.

The man in the bar. The man who ran into the bar had the hiccups. He asked for water to help get rid of them, but instead, the bartender pointed a gun at him. This frightened the man, which is another way to get rid of hiccups, and it worked. So the man thanked the bartender and left.

Test your powers of observation and memory, page 95

1. Skirt and blouse
2. Right
3. In her pocket
4. Blond
5. No
6. The mother
7. Doll
8. Child's hair
9. Sitting in a chair
10. Comb, hand mirror, box

Scoring:

9 - 10   Excellent observation and memory
7 - 8   Pretty sharp
5 - 6   Not too bad
1 - 4   Not so hot. It might help to look a little closer next time.
And to boost your memory, practice the tips in the *Memory* chapter.

Candle-mounting problem, page 108

Solving this problem requires recognizing that a box need not always serve as a container.

Trivia quiz, pages 108-109

1. uncopyrightable

2. Maine

3. False. You'll lose only about one-fifth of your vision but all of your depth perception.

4. Fleas, as carriers of the bubonic plague, have led to more human deaths. In fact, they have led to more loss of life than all the wars ever fought.

5. According to one survey, it's not breakfast, which about 9 percent of the population skips. It's lunch. On any given day about 22 percent miss that meal.

6. Men are more likely than women — and even more so if they are single — to flash a warning to oncoming traffic.

7. Alligators have a broader, rounder snout. And as to the tears, crocodiles have no tear ducts, so they can't shed real tears. But since they live predominantly in salt water marshes, they need the tear-like hormonal secretions to wash the harsh salt water from their eyes.

8. The car muffler

9. They take an equal amount of time.

10. Panama, due to a bend in the isthmus.

11. It contains a slice of moon rock.

12. On a child's second birthday, his height is approximately one-half his final height.

13. Thumbs up for the thumb. It uses more "gray matter" than the other two combined.

14. Hardwoods, like ash, oak, and beech, give off the most heat. Cherry is less efficient, and poplar the least desirable.

15. They lose their gold color. The same thing happens if you put them in dim light.

Measuring with 3 jugs, page 124

All seven problems can be solved by filling up jug B, then pouring out enough to fill jug A once and jug C two times.

First problem:

127 cups – 27 cups (21 cups + 3 cups + 3 cups) = 100 cups

Once you saw that every problem worked out the same way, you probably continued doing them all the same. Psychologists call that a mental set. But more flexible thinking would come in handy if you were actually pouring the water.

You'd save time on problems six and seven with a different solution. In problem six, you could fill jug A (23 cups) and pour out three cups to fill jug C, leaving 20 cups.

In problem seven, simply fill jug A and jug B for a total of 18 cups.

The illustrations below show problem one and problem six.

Problem 1   **Problem 6**

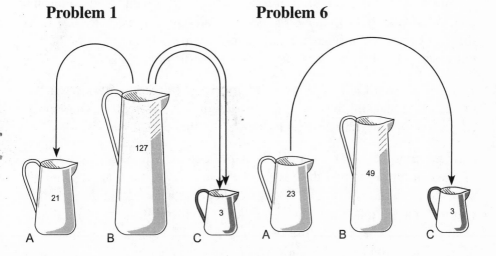

Syllabaloo, page 125

1. millennium
2. gigantic
3. cardinal
4. follow
5. pineapple
6. observation
7. peculiar
8. equipment
9. cardiologist
10. thanksgiving

Your 'write' personality, pages 135-136

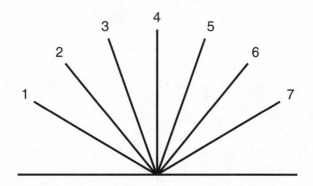

Slant — Slant 4 is a sign of a balanced person with good emotional control. Slants 5 to 7 indicate that you are an outgoing person who looks forward to new experiences. Slants 1 to 3 are usually people who have a tendency to be shy and hold back. They may dislike change.

Size — Small letters show a detail-oriented person with a talent for organizing facts and figures. Large letters indicate a creative, free-spirited person who doesn't like being tied to a schedule.

The capital I — If the capital "I" at the beginning of the sentence is simple and in proportion to the rest of the sentence, you are an easy-going, down-to-earth person. If your "I" is much larger than the rest of the sentence, you may have a touch of vanity and like to perform. If your "I" is tall and skinny, you have a great sense of family pride. If your "I" is written with straight lines, you are a straightforward, ambitious person.

The small i — If your small "i" in the word "personality" has a small dot above it, you are probably a careful person who is always on time for appointments. If you have a dark, heavy dot above your "i," you are positive and self-assured. If you have a little circle above your "i," you like beautiful things and enjoy being creative. If you have a dash high above the "i," you are an enthusiastic, adventurous person.

Now go back and try part two before you look at these answers.

1. For this position, you'd want someone outgoing and friendly — like Paula. Notice her large letters, especially the "I," with flourishes and open loops, written in a firm hand with letters flowing softly from left to right. These are characteristics of an extrovert.

On the other hand, Angie shows the qualities of an introvert — small, tight letters; writing with light pressure; and retracing lines rather than making loops in the stems of letters like "d" and "h." Definitely not your party girl.

2. Watch out for Morris! The unstable slant of his letters indicates an unpredictable, undisciplined individual. This and the "felon's claw" on the letter "I" are characteristic of the writing of 70 to 80 percent of all convicted criminals.

Furthermore, are you even sure what price he's offering? Embezzlers commonly write numbers illegibly, like the number 8 which might be taken for the number 5. They also prefer to write in pencil.

One or two of these alone might not mean you wouldn't get your money. But putting it all together, you'd best sell the vase to Harry.

3. Becky slows down to print "love," a word she may be hesitant to write. She may say it's in caps for emphasis, but the backward slant makes that doubtful.

4. Bearing down so much harder when writing her name could mean the writer feels quite frustrated with Agnes.

Attitude cryptograms, page 151

1. Nothing is good or bad but thinking makes it so. — William Shakespeare

2. What you see and hear depends a good deal on where you are standing; it also depends on what sort of person you are. — C. S. Lewis

3. The greater part of our happiness or misery depends on our dispositions and not our circumstances. — Martha Washington

4. You can complain because roses have thorns, or you can rejoice because thorns have roses. — Ziggy

5. The eye sees only what the mind is prepared to comprehend. — Henri Bergson

6. Re-examine all you have been told . . . Dismiss what insults your soul. — Walt Whitman

Awareness check, page 174

A. A total of 30 squares can be found. You probably picked out the 16 small squares without a problem. And you may have counted the 17th — the largest one — on the outside perimeter. That's where most people stop. But if you're a careful observer, you'll also see nine additional 2x2-inch squares and four 3x3-inch squares.

B. You probably read, "What is the point?" That seems simple, but it is not what it says. If you go back, you'll see that "the" appears twice. Fewer than 10 percent of readers are aware of the duplication.

C. Finding the "F's" is a challenge. There are nine, but most people find three to five because they miss those in the title or the word "of."

D. This is the toughest challenge for most people because they focus on the black designs and miss the white space in between. Try rotating the book clockwise a quarter turn and focus on the white space. You should see the word "FLY" in large block letters.

Happiness quiz, page 198

Questions one and two have no bearing on happiness. Research shows equal happiness across all ages, nationalities, and gender groups.

Happy people tend to answer yes to numbers three, four, five, and six.

Questions seven, eight, and nine are unrelated to happiness. But since happy people tend to see themselves as above average in most respects, whether it's based on fact or not, they might be more likely to answer yes to questions seven and nine as well.

Do you expect question 10 to require a yes answer? It could be yes or no. Many people who had unhappy childhoods find their adult life much better — to their great pleasure. And what about question 11? If you answered yes, you are typical of many happy people. You are likely to see today's happiness as greater when you compare it to times of unhappiness in the past.

Most happy people tend to be physically active, socially outgoing, and helpful to others. So for questions 12 through 16, they might choose taking a walk, gardening, talking to a friend, collecting for charity, and going to a party.

Rhyming pairs, page 199

1. Laurel and Hardy — comedians
2. Sonny and Cher — singers
3. Cain and Abel — biblical brothers
4. Tom and Jerry— cartoon rivals
5. Jan and Dean — singers
6. Dick and Jane — early reader characters
7. Mickey and Minnie — Disney characters
8. Roy (Rogers) and Dale (Evans) — singing western actors
9. Adam and Eve — biblical characters
10. Beauty and the Beast — fairy tale characters

Bedtime logic problem, pages 219-221

Name	Profession	Pajamas	Bedtime
Knight	politician	wild animals	12:30
Dozzer	actor	candy stripes	10:30
Napper	dancer	polka dots	11:30
Nodder	ice skater	teddy bears	1:00
Shuteye	singer	tartan plaid	11:00

Fun facts dream quiz, page 239

1. False. REM is found in young birds as well.

2. True. Females dream about males and females equally. But in males' dreams, about 65 percent of the time the other characters are also male.

3. False. This myth has been around a long time, but plenty of people have dreamed it and lived to tell about it. There's also the myth that if you dream you die, you will. It is also false. Some people who study the meanings of dreams believe that a dream of death is more likely to indicate the end of something old and the beginning of something new.

4. False. Each dreamer has his or her own dream symbols. What a house means to one can be very different from what it means to another person. But dreams can give clues to things that are happening with your health, sometimes before you have consciously noticed.

5. False. "Frequent fliers" tend to be more self-confident and optimistic than more "grounded" dreamers.

6. True. Einstein's dreams, for example, gave him the symbols with which to explain the principles of relativity. Artists Salvadore Dali

and Henri Rousseau got images for some of their paintings from their dreams. Steve Allen found lines for one of his most popular songs, *This Could be the Start of Something Big*, in a dream.

7. True. First-born females dream more about aggressive strangers, while middle females (with at least one older and one younger sibling) find friendlier folk in their dreams. Last-borns dream less often about babies and children.

8. True — although you may not be aware of color in remembering your dreams. Women remember color more often than men. If you are especially aware of tints and hues when you are awake, you will probably notice them more in dreams. The emotional intensity of the dream may be indicated by the depth and brightness of the colors.

9. False. Even people who spend most of their day doing these tasks rarely dream about them. But activities like walking, talking with friends, and having sex are common.

10. True. While the average adult spends an hour and a half in REM sleep each night, a newborn may spend as much as nine hours in REM. What do you suppose the dreams are about? Perhaps they are pleasant dreams. A baby's first "smile" usually occurs during REM sleep.

All hands on deck!, page 254

If you got them all right, you are captain of your brain's ship. If you missed only one or two, you should be named first mate. Four or less, you need to drop anchor and think some more.

1. Worship	5. Friendship	9. Craftsmanship
2. Kinship	6. Township	10. Salesmanship
3. Scholarship	7. Citizenship	11. Championship
4. Hardship	8. Leadership	12. Ownership

Mental mix-up, page 278

esridpsnoe	depression	odom	mood
zcrapo	prozac	sgemasa	massage
cxeesrei	exercise	setsrs	stress
ionasmin	insomnia	xeitnay	anxiety
erhat esadies	heart disease	eatihpstr	therapist
trohpmyhidsiyo	hypothyroidism	ts hjosn rowt	st johns wort
odlob srespuer	blood pressure		
stiumrnosentrtane	neurotransmitters		

naselaso eftavfcie sedorrid   seasonal affective disorder

It's all in your head, pages 292-293

1. Heads or tails
2. Bullheaded
3. Headlights
4. Headless horseman
5. Head over heels
6. Don't let your head rule your heart

Word search, page 310

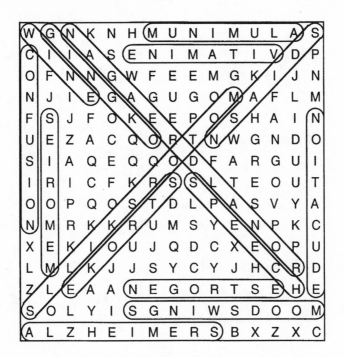

High-ho, page 323

1. high chair

2. come hell or high water

3. high tail

4. high noon

5. thigh

6. high heels

7. high five

8. high jinks

9. highlight

10. knee high

What's the difference?, pages 324-325

Cup:

Coffee in cup.

Extra rose leaf.

Dashed line on plate.

Cup handles are different.

Veins missing from rose leaf.

Flower design on teacup is reversed.

Flowers and basket:

Bigger shadow beneath basket.

Ladybug on basket handle.

Flower missing on left side.

Several threads missing on basket handle.

Find the Foods word search, pages 344-345

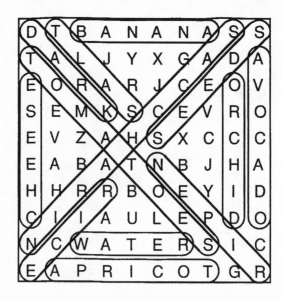

Observation and Memory picture, page 95

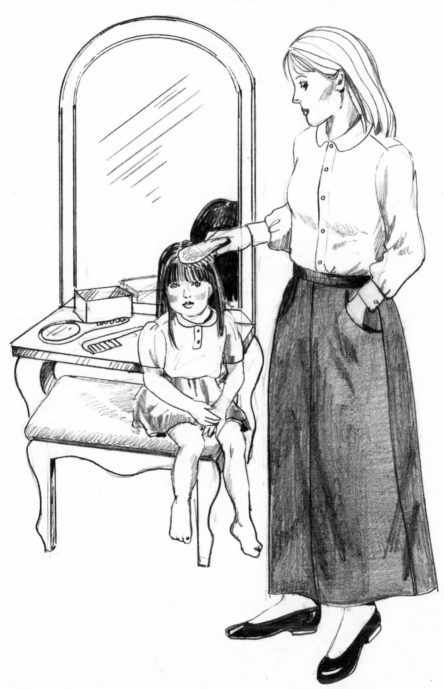

Sources

Alzheimer's

Alzheimer's Disease, Publication No. 94-3676, National Institutes of Health, Bethesda, MD 20892

Alzheimer's Disease: An Update <www.medscape.com/quadrant/Hospital Medicine/1997/v33.n10/hm3310.01/> retrieved Dec. 8, 1997

American Journal of Epidemiology (139,1:48)

Archives of Neurology (53,9:922)

Estrogen Replacement Therapy Reduces Risk of Alzheimer's Disease by 54 percent, American Academy of Neurology <www.aan.com/public_xls/nr15estro-gen2.htm> retrieved Oct. 21, 1997

Geriatrics (34,17:21)

Griffith's 5 Minute Consultant, Williams & Wilkins, Baltimore, Md., 1996

Is it Alzheimer's? Warning Signs You Should Know, Alzheimer's Association, 919 North Michigan Ave., Suite 1000, Chicago, IL 60611

Medical Tribune for the Internist and Cardiologist (35,16:8; 35,4:14; and 36,20:19)

Naturwissenschaften (84:1)

Neurology (45:51 and 46:641)

Revue Neurologique (153,3:185)

Science News (150,10:154 and 150,25&26:399)

Scientific American <www.sciam.com/0696issue/0696scic-it08.html> retrieved Dec. 11, 1997

Smoking Increases the Risk of Dementia, American Academy of Neurology <www.aan.com/public_xls/nr08demen-tia2.htm> retrieved Oct. 21, 1997

Super Lifespan, Super Health, FC&A Publishing, Peachtree City, Ga., 1997

The American Medical Association Encyclopedia of Medicine, Random House, New York, 1989

The Journal of the American Medical Association (271,13:1004; 275,7:528; 275,18:1389; 277,10:813; 278,16:1327; and 283,8:1007,1055)

The Lancet (342,8874:793; 345,8963:1481; and 347,9001:573)

The New England Journal of Medicine (336,17:1216)

Attitude

American Heart Journal (132,6:1207)

Annual Review of Medicine 1996 (47:193)

British Medical Journal (310,6971:70)

Cultivating a Positive Attitude, M.J. Gimeno, M.D. <www.Altnewtimes.com> retrieved May 1, 1998

Emotion and Motivation, National Institute of Mental Health <www.nimh.nih.gov> retrieved April 16, 1998

Feeling Good: The New Mood Therapy, Avon Books, New York, 1992

Journal of Psychosomatic Research (47,3:241)

Managing Your Mind: The Mental Fitness Guide, Oxford University Press, New York, 1996

Mind/Body Health, Allyn and Bacon, Boston, 1996

Psychology, Worth Publishers, New York, 1995

Self-Esteem, New Harbinger Publications, Inc., Oakland, Calif., 1992

What is Cognitive Therapy? Robert Westermeyer, Ph.D. <www.cts.com> retrieved April 1, 1998

Working With Self-Esteem in Psychotherapy, Nathaniel Brandon, Ph.D. <www.vix.com> retrieved Nov. 4, 1997

Creativity

Arts in Psychotherapy (8,3-4:185)

British Journal of Sports Medicine (31,3:240)

Creativity: Beyond the Myth of Genius, W.H. Freeman and Co., New York, 1993

Forced Analogy <www.ozemail. com.au/~caveman/Creative/Techniques/ forced_analogy.htm> retrieved Oct. 15, 1997

Indian Psychological Review (28,5:5)

Mind Maps <www.ozemail. com.au/~caveman/Creative/Mindmap/in dex.htm> retrieved Oct. 15, 1997

Problem Reversal <www.ozemail. com.au/~caveman/Creative/Techniques/ reversal.htm> retrieved Oct. 15, 1997

Psychological Reports (71,1:43)

Random Input <www.ozemail. com.au/~caveman/Creative/Techniques/ random.htm> retrieved Oct. 15, 1997

Science News (147,24:378)

Scientific American (272,2:62)

Six Thinking Hats <www.ozemail. com.au/~caveman/Creative/Techniques/ sixhats.htm> retrieved Oct. 15, 1997

Depression

801 Prescription Drugs: Good Effects, Side Effects & Natural Healing Alternatives, FC&A Publishing, Peachtree City, Ga., 1996

Alternative and Complementary Therapies (2,1:1)

American Psychologist (52,1:25)

Annals of Medicine (25,4:301)

Archives of Family Medicine (6,1:43)

Archives of General Psychiatry (54,10:915 and 56,5:407)

Arthritis Today (9,6:9)

British Medical Journal (313,7052:253)

Circulation (93,11:1976 and 102,18:2296)

Comprehensive Psychiatry (38,2:80 and 38,5:289)

Consumer Reports (60,11:734)

Depression Linked to Bone Loss, National Institute of Mental Health <www.nimh.nih.gov/events/prbones.htm> retrieved Sept. 8, 2000

Diabetes in the News (13,6:32)

Dr. Joseph Hibbeln, Laboratory of Membrane Biophysics and Biochemistry, NIAAA, National Institutes of Health, Bethesda, Md.

Dr. William Lands, Senior Advisor, NIAAA, National Institutes of Health, Bethesda, Md.

Eicosanoid formation, receptor functions, and clinical relevance, Paper presented at: Essential Fats In Foods workshop; March 20, 2000; Bethesda, Md.

Finding Help: How to Choose a Psychologist, American Psychological Association <www.apa.org/pubinfo/howto.html> retrieved Sept. 8, 2000

Herbal Prescriptions for Better Health, Prima Publishing, Rocklin, Ca., 1996

Herbs for Health (1,3:51)

International Journal of Clinical Practice (54,1:57)

Journal of Affective Disorders (48,2-3:149)

Keep It Managed, National Institutes of Health <http://intramural.niaaa.nih.gov/eicosanoids> retrieved Nov. 1, 2000

Lipids (31, Suppl:S163)

McLean Hospital news release (May 13, 1999)

Millions with "the blues" may actually have thyroid disease, American Association of Clinical Endocrinologists <www.aace.com> retrieved Sept. 8, 2000

Neuroreport (6,14:1853)

New Statesman (Sept. 20, 1999)

Nihon Shinkei Seishin Yakurigaku Zasshi (15,1:39)

Omega 6 and omega 3 fatty acid content of common foods <http://gemini.oscs.montana.edu/~bchem280/omega.html> retrieved Nov. 3, 2000

Omega-3 Oils: A Practical Guide, Avery Publishing Group, Garden City Park, N.Y., 1996

Plain Talk About... Depression, Publication No. (ADM) 92-1639, National Institute of Mental Health, 5600 Fishers Lane, Rockville, MD 20857

Psychology, Worth Publishers, New York, 1995

Science (279,5349:396)

The American Medical Association Family Medical Guide, Random House, New York, 1994

The Health Answer Book: The Complete Guide to Symptoms, Causes, and Natural Cures for Hundreds of Health Problems, FC&A Publishing, Peachtree City, Ga., 1997

The Lancet (351,9110:1213)

The Omega Diet, HarperCollins, New York, 1999

The Physician and Sportsmedicine (23,9:44)

Dreaming

British Medical Journal (306,6883:993)

Common Questions about Dreams, Association for the Study of Dreams <www.ASDreams.org/commque.html> retrieved Oct. 9, 1997

Common Questions About Nightmares, Association for the Study of Dreams <www.asdreams.org/nightma.htm> retrieved Feb. 5, 1998

Dreaming (6,2:1)

Exploring the World of Lucid Dreaming, Ballantine, New York, 1990

Getting More REM Sleep Contributes to Waking Up in a Good Mood, Center for Sleep and Stress <www.quantadynamics.com/css/qreportjuly97-03.htm> retrieved Feb. 13, 1998

In Your Dreams, Harper, San Francisco, 1997

Journal of Behavior Therapy and Experimental Psychiatry (24,4:325)

Journal of the Association for the Study of Dreams (1,4:277)

Lucid Dreaming, Ballantine, New York, 1985

Lucid Dreaming Frequently Asked Questions and Answers, The Lucidity Institute <www.lucidity.com/LucidDreamingFAQ2.html> retrieved March 10, 1997

Our Dreaming Mind, Ballantine, New York, 1994

Psychology, Worth Publishers, New York, 1995

The Brain, Lucent Books, Inc., San Diego, 1996

The Enchanted World of Sleep, Yale University Press, New Haven, 1996

Where People Fly and Water Runs Uphill, Warner Books, New York, 1992

Working (and playing) with Dreams, John Suler, Ph.D. <www1.rider.edu/~suler/dreams.html#FreeWriting> retrieved Feb. 4, 1998

Emotions

American Behavioral Scientist (39,3:249)

Arthritis Today (5,5:44)

Catheterization and Cardiovascular Diagnosis (42,2:242)

Clinical Psychiatric News (25,6:15)

Color Research and Application (22,2:121,448)

Compendium of Olfactory Research 1982-1994, Kendall/Hunt Publishing, Dubuque, Iowa, 1995

Coping with Loss – Bereavement and Grief, National Mental Health Association <www.nmha.org> retrieved Dec. 1, 1997

Current Health 2 (22,4:26)

Emotions and Motivation, National Institute of Mental Health <www.nimh.nih.gov/publicatbaschap1.htm#box1> retrieved April 16, 1998

European Journal of Cancer Care (4,1:17)

Health Psychology (14,4:341)

Healthy Pleasures, Addison-Wesley Publishing Company, Inc., Reading, Mass., 1989

Holiday Cards Really Do Spread Cheer, Study Says, Penn State University <www.eurekalert.org:80/release/psu-hdcdsc.html> retrieved Dec. 15, 1997

Holistic Nurse Practitioner (10,2:49)

Journal of Behavioral Medicine (20,1:29)

Journal of Personality and Social Psychology (73,4:687)

The Journal of the American Medical Association (277,24:1940)

Journal of the National Cancer Institute (87,5:342)

Laughter as Therapy for Patient and Caregiver, Patty Wooten, R.N. <www.jestforhealth.com/ch_pulm.html> retrieved Aug. 2, 2000

Medical Tribune (36,14:20)

Mind/Body Health, Allyn and Bacon, Boston, 1996

Mothering (62,52:6)

Psychological Science (7,3:181)

Psychology, Worth Publishers, New York, 1995

Psychology Today (29,4:32)

Right Side of the Brain Does the Work for Worriers, Johns Hopkins Medical Institution <www.eurekalert.org:80/releases/right-side-worriers.html> retrieved Oct. 28, 1997

Risk Factors Cluster to Harm Health, National Institutes of Health <www1.od.nih.gov/obssr/riskclu.htm> retrieved Dec. 1, 1997

Road Rage – How to Avoid Aggressive Driving, Corporate Facts and Announcements – AAA Foundation for Traffic Safety Brochure <www.aaa-calif.com/members/corpinforoadrage.htm> retrieved April 17, 1998

Socialization – Not Just Genes – Is What Makes Men Tick and May Make Them Sick, American Psychological Association <www.apa.org/releases/socializ.html> retrieved Dec. 1, 1997

The Happiness Problem, Rasmussen Research <www.portraitofamerica.com/releases/1097102897b.htm> retrieved April 2, 1998

The Importance of Understanding Loneliness, Perspectives: A Mental Health Magazine <www.cmhc.com/perspectives/ articles/art09963.htm> retrieved October 21, 1997

The Phases and Tasks of Grief Work, Self-Help and Psychology Magazine <www.shpm.com/articles/loss/phases.html> retrieved August 2, 2000

The Review of Natural Products, Facts and Comparisons, St. Louis, Mo.

The Structure of Emotion, National Institute of Mental Health <www.nimh.nih.gov/publicat/basbox1.htm> retrieved April 16, 1998

American Heart Association news release (Nov. 10, 1997)

Headache

Feverfew, American Botanical Council, Austin, Texas, 1996

Headache, Supplement to Mayo Clinic Health Letter (October 1993)

Migraine, Tension and Cluster Headaches <www.aafp.org/patientinfo/headache.html> retrieved Nov. 4, 1997

NHF Headlines (Spring 1996 and Winter 1998)

Postgraduate Medicine (98,2:197)

The Lancet (348,9042:1649)

The Newnan Times-Herald (May 8, 1996, 4B)

Inside your brain

Psychology, Worth Publishers, New York, 1995

Psychology Today (30,4:11)

The American Medical Association Encyclopedia of Medicine, Random House, New York, 1989

Intelligence

Acta Psychiatrica Scandinavica (81,3:265)

American Psychologist (52,7:685)

Ceska A Slovenska Oftalmologie (51,4:235)

Emotional Intelligence, Bantam Books, New York, 1995

FDA Consumer (26,4:3)

Frames of Mind: The Theory of Multiple Intelligences, BasicBooks, New York, 1993

Governor proposes infant music giveaway <www.my.excite.com/news/r/980113/17/odd-music> retrieved Jan. 14, 1998

Health and Stress (7:1)

Inside the Brain, Andrews and McMeel, Kansas City, Mo., 1996

Journal of Personality and Social Psychology (36,1:1)

Multiple Intelligence Key <www.athena.ivv.nasa.gov/curric/land/wetland/multint.html> retrieved Jan. 30, 1998

Multiple Intelligence Theory <www.scbe.on.ca/mit/mi.htm#DEF> retrieved Jan. 30, 1998

Nature (383,6602:670)

Neurology (41,5:644)

Neuroscience Letters (185,1:44)

Psychology Today (30,1:18)

Psychology, Worth Publishers, New York, 1995

Psychophysiology (31,6:525)

Seven Ways of Knowing: Teaching for Multiple Intelligences <www.iriskylight.com/SevenWK/swoki.htm> retrieved Jan. 30, 1998

Super Lifespan Super Health, FC&A, Peachtree City, Ga., 1997

Introduction

Neuroscience, Memory and Language, Library of Congress, Washington, 1995

Proceedings of the National Academy of Sciences (95,6:3168)

Update 1998: Reshaping Expectations, The Dana Press, New York, 1998

Learning

A Client's Feedback on Brain Gym and NLP, The ADD Action Group <www.addgroup.org/braingym.htm.> retrieved April 16, 1998

About Brain Gym <www.users.aol/braingym/bg.html> retrieved April 16, 1998

American Journal of Epidemiology (130,5:999)

Brain Building in Just 12 Weeks, Bantam Books, New York, 1990

Double Your Brain Power, Prentice Hall, Paramus, N.J., 1997

Managing Your Mind — The Mental Fitness Guide, Oxford University Press, New York, 1995

Nature (386,6624:493)

Ruth Upchurch, Instructor, Brain Gym, Atlanta, Ga.

Male vs. female

Scientific American (267,3:119)

Sex on the Brain, Viking, New York, 1997

The Economist (338,7954:85)

The Lancet (351,9102:575)

Memory

801 Prescription Drugs, FC&A Publishing, Peachtree City, Ga., 1996

American Journal of Epidemiology (144,3:275; 145,1:33; and 145,6:507)

Archives of Internal Medicine (156,19:2213)

Health and Stress: The Newsletter of the American Institute of Stress (7:1)

Journal of Cognitive Neuroscience (9,5:555)

Journal of the American College of Nutrition (15,6:630)

Medical Tribune for Internists and Cardiologists (37,17:16)

Psychology, Worth Publishers, New York, 1995

Science (276,5313:675)

Scientists Find Testosterone Supplements Improve Working Memory in Older Men, Oregon Health Sciences University <www.eurekalert.org:80/releases/test-epi-tox.html> retrieved Oct. 28, 1997

Super Lifespan Super Health, FC&A, Peachtree City, Ga., 1997

The American Journal of Clinical Nutrition (61,4S:987S)

The American Medical Association Encyclopedia of Medicine, Random House, New York, 1989

The Guardian (Feb. 11, 1997)

The Health Answer Book, FC&A Publishing, Peachtree City, Ga., 1997

Mindpower

Alternative Medicine: Expanding Medical Horizons, Report to the National Institutes of Health, Sept. 14-16, 1992

Alternative Therapies (4,1:75 and 4,2:32)

American Family Physician (50,5:1067)

American Journal of Cardiology (77,10:867)

Behavior Research and Therapy (33,2:145)

Job Stress Reduction Therapies <www.healthonline.com > retrieved Nov. 13, 1997

Journal of Behavior Therapy and Experimental Psychiatry (26,1:1)

Journal of Criminal Justice (15,3:211)

Journal of Holistic Nursing (13,3:255)

Journal of Personality and Social Psychology (57,6:950)

Nurse Practitioner (22,3:150)

Nursing Clinics of North America (30,4:697)

Opthalmologica (209,3:122)

Proceedings of the National Academy of Sciences (95,6:3168)

Psychological Reports (76,3:929 and 77,2:403)

Psychosomatic Medicine (57:177)

Psychotherapy and Psychosomatics (66,4:185)

Science (273,5276:749)

The American Holistic Health Association's Complete Guide to Alternative Medicine, Warner Books, 1996

The Mind/Heart Connection, William Collinge, Ph.D. <www.healthy.net/collinge/heart.htm> retrieved Feb. 26, 1998

The Three Minute Meditator, New Harbinger Publications, Oakland, Calif., 1996

Timeless Healing, Scribner, New York, 1996

What is Biofeedback?, DHHS Publication No. (ADM) 83-1273, U.S. Department of Health and Human Services, 1983

Nutrition

Archives of Family Medicine (4,4:304)

Archives of General Psychiatry (54,6:537)

Archives of Pediatric and Adolescent Medicine (150:1089)

British Medical Journal (312,7043:1378)

Choose a Diet With Plenty of Vegetables, Fruits, and Grain Products, United States Department of Agriculture, Home and Garden Bulletin Number 253-5, Washington, 1993

Environmental Health Perspectives (102,7S:65)

Environmental Nutrition (19,12:7)

FDA Warns Against Drug Promotion of "Herbal Fen-Phen," Food and Drug Administration, U.S. Department of Health and Human Services, Rockville, Md., 1997

Hamilton and Whitney's Nutrition Concepts and Controversies, West Publishing Co., St. Paul, Minn., 1994

Headache (37,10:654)

Journal of Nutrition (125,6:1484 and 125,8S:2263)

Journal of the American College of Nutrition (19,2:207,242)

Lon R. White, M.D., Pacific Health Research Institute

Methods and Findings in Experimental and Clinical Pharmacology (17,SupplB:2 and 19,3:201)

National Institute of Mental Health press release (Aug. 26, 1997)

Nature (382:677)

Nutrition Almanac, McGraw-Hill, New York, 1996

Nutritional Intervention in the Aging Process, Springer-Verlag, Inc., New York, 1984

Pharmacy Times (62,12:84)

Potatoes Not Prozac, Simon & Schuster, New York, 1998

Psychology Today (29,3:34 and 30,6:14)

Shape Up America General Information <www2.shapeup.org/sua/general/index. html> retrieved on April 29, 1998

Super Lifespan, Super Health, FC&A Publishing, Peachtree City, Ga., 1997

The Big Book of Health Tips, FC&A Publishing, Peachtree City, Ga., 1996

The Columbia University College of Physicians and Surgeons Complete Home Medical Guide, Crown Publishers, 1989

Personality

Cornell University news release (Oct. 15, 1996)

Journal of Personality and Social Psychology (65,1:176)

Journal of Personality Assessment (69,1:104)

Mind/Body Health, Allyn and Bacon, Boston, 1996

Nature Genetics (12,1:81)

Overcoming Procrastination: A New Look, William J. Knzus, Ed.D. <rebt.org/essays/procrst1.htm> retrieved May 4, 1998

Perceptual and Motor Skills (81,2:1203)

Science News (150,10:154)

The Healing Brain: A Scientific Reader, The Guilford Press, New York, 1990

Sharper thinking

Critical Thinking - Evaluating Claims and Arguments in Everyday Life, Mayfield Publishing Co., Palo Alto, Calif., 1986

Managing Your Mind, Oxford University Press, New York, 1995

Overcoming Procrastination: A New Look, <www.iret.org/essays/procrst1.html> retrieved Dec. 3, 1997

Overcoming Procrastination: Part II <www.iret.org/essays/procrst2.html> retrieved Dec. 3, 1997

Paul Sloane's List of Classic Lateral Thinking Puzzles <www.einstein.et.tudelft.nV-ariet/puzzles/lateral.html> retrieved Oct. 8, 1997

Serious Creativity: Using the Power of Lateral Thinking to Create New Ideas, HarperBusiness, New York, 1992

The Directory for Building Competencies, Kravetz Associates, Bartlett, Ill., 1995

Think Out of the Box, Career Press, Franklin Lakes, N.J., 1997

Tne Big Book of Health Tips, FC&A Publishing, Peachtree City, Ga., 1996

Sleep

ABCs of ZZZs, National Sleep Foundation <www.websciences.org/nsf/publications/ZZZs.htm> retrieved Oct. 23, 1997

American Journal of Public Health (87,10:1649)

Canadian Medical Association Journal (154,8:1193)

Common Causes of Excessive Daytime Sleepiness, National Sleep Foundation <www.sleepfoundation.org/PressArchives/CommonCauses.htm> retrieved Dec. 24, 1997

Driver Sleepiness — "in-car" countermeasures: cold air and car radio, Loughborough University <www.websciences.org/cgi-shl/dbml.exe?Action=Query&Template=/APSS> retrieved Oct. 22, 1997

Facts About Drowsy Driving, National Sleep Foundation <www.websciences.org/nsf/activities/daaafacts.htm> retrieved Nov. 20, 1997

Facts about insomnia, Publication No. 95-3801, National Institutes of Health, Bethesda, MD 20824

Journal of Psychosomatic Research (42,6:583)

Nap time can be for the adults in the '90s workplace, Washington Post, 1997

Nature (379:540)

Neurology (48,4:904)

Peppermint aroma as a countermeasure to sleepiness during driving simulation, Institute for Circadian Physiology <www.websciences.org/cgi-shl/dbml.exe?Action=Query&Template=/APSS/> retrieved Oct. 22, 1997

Physiology and Behavior (60:681)

Sleep (19,4:318; 19,5:412; and 20,7:505)

Sleep and the Traveler, The National Sleep Foundation <www.sleepfoundation.org> retrieved Aug. 22, 2000

Sleep Research in the UK is Working Late, Britannia Internet Magazine <www.britannia.com/science/sleep.html> retrieved Dec. 24, 1997

Sleep Walking, Talking, Nightmares, Terrors & Eating, National Sleep Foundation <www.healthtouch.com/level1/leaflets/sleep/sleep006.htm> retrieved Oct. 28, 1997

Strategies for Shift Workers, National Sleep Foundation <www.sleepfoundation.org/publications/shiftworker.html> retrieved Jan. 14, 1998

The Big Book of Health Tips, FC&A, Peachtree City, Ga., 1996

The Enchanted World of Sleep, Yale University Press, New Haven, 1996

The Health Answer Book, FC&A Publishing, Peachtree City, Ga., 1997

The Lancet (346,8976:701 and 350,9091:1611)

The New England Journal of Medicine (334,14:924)

The Sciences (38,1:7)

U.S.Pharmacist (22,12:62)

Stroke

Age Page — Stroke: Prevention and Treatment, National Institute on Aging, U.S. Department of Health and Human Services, 1991

British Medical Journal (305,6867:1446 and 307,6898:231)

FDA Consumer (27,3:35)

Medical Tribune for the Internist and Cardiologist (36,16:5)

Science News (149,22:345)

Stroke (24,7:983; 29,1:159; 28,10:1919; and 31,6:1210)

The Atlanta Journal/Constitution (April 17, 1997, G3)

The Lancet (343,8899:687)

The Washington Post (Oct. 9, 1997)

U.S. Pharmacist (19,1:14)

Warning Signs of a Stroke, National
Institutes of Health, National Institute
of Neurological Disorders and Stroke,
Bethesda, Md.

Your aging brain

Inside the Brain, Andrews and McMeel,
Kansas City, 1996

Journal of Gerontology, Series B,
Psychological Science and Social
Sciences (52,6:294)

New Scientist (157,2118:10)

Omni (14,8:40)

Postgraduate Medicine (102,4:216)

Psychology, Worth Publishers, New York,
1995

Science News (152,11:174)

The Book of Lists, the '90s Edition, Little,
Brown and Company, Boston, 1993

Your divided brain

Doctor's Guide to Medical & Other News
<www.pslgroup.com/dg/4012e.htm>
retrieved Nov. 14, 1997

Left Brain, Right Brain, W.H. Freeman
and Co., New York, 1993

Postgraduate Medicine (102,6:144)

Psychology, Worth Publishers, New York,
1995

Science (259,5098:1118)

*The American Medical Association
Encyclopedia of Medicine*, Random
House, New York, 1989

The Right-Brain Experience, McGraw
Hill, New York, 1983

Index